DEVELOPMENTAL APRAXIA OF SPEECH

Developmental Apraxia of Speech

THEORY AND CLINICAL PRACTICE

Penelope K. Hall
Linda S. Jordan
Donald A. Robin

pro·ed
8700 Shoal Creek Boulevard
Austin, Texas 78757

Note. The authors, whose names are listed alphabetically, have the
following affiliations: Penelope K. Hall, MA, Department of
Speech Pathology and Audiology, University of Iowa; Linda S.
Jordan, PhD, Departments of Neurology, and Speech Pathology
and Audiology, University of Iowa; and Donald A. Robin, PhD,
Department of Speech Pathology and Audiology, and National
Center for Voice and Speech, University of Iowa. RJ496
.S7
H33
1993

Printed in the United States of America

Library of Congress Cataloging-in-Publication Data

Hall, Penelope K.
  Developmental apraxia of speech : theory and clinical practice /
Penelope K. Hall, Linda S. Jordan, Donald A. Robin.
    p.   cm.
  Includes bibliographic references and index.
  ISBN 0-89079-582-7
  1. Articulation disorders in children.   2. Apraxia.   I. Jordan.
Linda S.   II. Robin, Donald A.   III. Title.
RJ496.S7H33   1993
618.92′8552—dc20   92-42727
                                                              CIP

pro·ed
8700 Shoal Creek Boulevard
Austin, Texas 78757

  2   3   4   5   6   7   8   9   10   97   96   95   94

Contents

Preface

A Letter to Our Readers

Our purpose in writing this book is to share our view of developmental apraxia of speech (DAS) and our experiences working with this disorder. Readers will search in vain for a chapter that provides a formal presentation of diagnostic procedures. Instead we have included observations about procedures we find helpful in the diagnostic process. Readers will note the inclusion of assessment sections throughout the book following discussions of characteristics or issues related to DAS. A brief overview of the format of the book follows.

Chapter 1 introduces our background and philosophy about Developmental Apraxia of Speech. Chapter 2, "Speech Characteristics of Developmental Apraxia of Speech," introduces the reader to the methodological problems encountered in the study of the disorder and describes specific characteristics including speech sound errors and sequencing difficulties. Inconsistency and variability of errors as well as reports on intelligibility are also addressed. Finally, prognosis for response to treatment is reviewed.

A key feature in the presentation of the book's position is the appreciation of "Theories of Motor Control: Descriptions, Issues, and Potential for Explaining Developmental Apraxia of Speech" presented in chapter 3. Theories of motor control are illustrated. The potential offered by selected models for explanations of DAS is summarized.

DAS exists not in a vacuum, but in the context of the rest of the child's experiences. Therefore, we have addressed "Language and Academic Learning Problems: Co-occurring Characteristics of Children Exhibiting DAS" in chapter 4. Other co-occurring factors describing children with DAS are presented in chapter 5, "Familial and Genetic Factors," which highlights familial history, DAS in syndromes, and sex rations; and Chapter 6, "Neurologic and Psychologic Factors."

Chapters 7, 8, and 9 illustrate our views on remediation techniques for children with DAS. Chapter 7 presents "Remediation: Motor Programming Approaches to Developmental Apraxia of Speech." Chapter 8, "Remediation: Specific Remedial Techniques," describes methods we believe to be compatible with our overall approach to treatment of children with DAS. Chapter 9 presents "Remediation: Specific Issues Associated With the Communication Remediation of Children With DAS."

We are obviously excited about this topic, but the future is yours. Chapter 10 is not intended to give you, the readers, future direction, but invites you to investigate and contribute to the knowledge base of developmental apraxia of speech. To close, we have attempted to share as extensive a bibliography as reasonably possible so that you can take advantage of the library work we have done. The majority of these references are reviewed in the text; the remainder are included for the sake of completeness.

Acknowledgments

We would like to acknowledge Margie Watkinson for her secretarial support throughout the evolution of this text. Her attention to detail and timely efficiency greatly facilitated our efforts. Her involvement in and devotion to the project are deeply appreciated.

We wish to acknowledge the children with DAS and their parents who have motivated us to study this disorder. We would also like to acknowledge our graduate students with whom we have interacted in the clinic, in our own research programs, and in discussions about DAS. These have all furthered the development of our ideas.

Finally, we are grateful for the process of sharing with each other, and with you, the readers. This process has encouraged us to dig deeper into the literature and into our thinking. Here we share with you the results of these efforts.

P.K.H.
L.S.J.
D.A.R.

CHAPTER I

Introduction
and Philosophy

The authors (hereafter referred to as "we") work in a facility where, in addition to serving community needs, we serve as consultants in a statewide capacity to clinicians who seek second opinions and assistance in their clinical efforts with specific children. Hadden (1891) described an 11-year-old with such severe compromise of speech sound production that "even the simplest words, such as 'cat', could not be rendered so as to be recognized by others. When he talked or read [aloud] it was evident that he was dividing off into syllables, although the sounds were unintelligible gibberish" (p. 97). If this child, Charles M., happened into our clinic, he would, except for wardrobe, fit comfortably with the group we describe as exhibiting *developmental apraxia of speech* (DAS).

Many referrals of children with DAS to our clinic are generated because the referring clinicians do not feel quite adequate to the child's obvious communication needs. We are sympathetic to these clinicians' requests because our own growth in understanding the DAS population has been fostered by the opportunity to work with a number of these children whose original remedial programs had been devised by numerous clinicians from a large geographic area.

Because we work in close proximity to each other in a research and clinical environment, we are repeatedly drawn together to test our observations and conclusions. As with other clinicians, our concept of ourselves as clinicians and our knowledge of what we can accomplish is reinforced with every goal that is set and met. Our growth as clinicians is perhaps defined by unmet goals that have forced us to revise our knowledge base and attempt innovative approaches. We recognize the relatively unique opportunity we have been afforded and have chosen to share through this book our current state of clinical experience with children exhibiting DAS.

For many speech clinicians who work with children to improve speech sound production, there stands out in their memory at least one child with normal hearing who did not make progress at the anticipated rate, despite the clinician's best efforts, the child's cooperation, and the family's support. The child's use of facial expressions, gestures, non-speech sounds, and isolated words or social phrases with which communicative success could be guaranteed, assured the clinician that the child wanted to communicate. No apparent structural impairment or paralysis of the oral mechanism explained the absence of intelligible speech. Auditory comprehension skills appeared to be adequate to support communication. Past success with children who had what appeared to be equally severely impoverished communication skills indicated that the clinician possessed the clinical skills necessary to develop or implement remediation programs that had proven successful with the majority of clients. Nevertheless, with this child such success was not demonstrated.

The clinician may have referred the child to other specialists and tested with a variety of instruments in an attempt to discover the key to unlock the mystery and explain the child's lack of successful response to clinical efforts. Over the years, the clinician watched in frustration as the child slipped into a non-communicative mode, unable to control the environment through verbal means. Frustration may have been shared as a different clinician took over the remedial effort or as counsel was sought from other clinicians. With increasing awareness of a number of such children, the profession as a whole sought solutions in group meetings and discussions. Some chose to embrace new terms such as *developmental motor aphasia* (Orton, 1937); *executive aphasia* (Worster-Draught, 1953); *articulatory apraxia* (Morley, Court, & Miller, 1954); *innervatory apraxia* (McGinnis, 1963); *congenital articulatory apraxia* (Eisenson, 1972); *developmental apraxia of speech* (Rosenbek & Wertz, 1972); *developmental verbal apraxia* (Edwards, 1973); *dilapidated speech* (Ferry, Hall, & Hicks, 1975); and *phonologic programming deficit syndrome* (Rapin & Allen, 1981). These labels gave us the confidence that, if nothing else had been achieved, at least the diagnosis was recognized. Surely the approach to remediation would soon be developed. Comforting too, perhaps, was the knowledge that with the diagnosis came the explanation for failure—these children were known to make slow progress in treatment (Morley et al., 1954; Ferry et al., 1975; Aram & Glasson, 1979).

Use of the Term *Apraxia* to Describe a Developmental Problem

Many of the aforementioned labels incorporate the term *apraxia*. Some individuals oppose the diagnosis of apraxia of speech in children because they theoretically disagree with the explanation for the disorder implied by the use of the term. ''Some authors are reluctant to associate the term apraxia with a speech disorder unless a skill has been lost thus rejecting the concept of developmental apraxia,'' (Bernthal & Bankson, 1988, p. 174).

We have no objections to the use of the term *apraxia* to describe the developmental speech problems of some children. Apraxia has traditionally been described as an inability to produce purposeful movements in the absence of paralysis, sensory impairments, comprehension problems, or intellectual disorders (Liepmann, 1900). In the adult, acquired apraxia of speech usually occurs as a result of a lesion to Broca's area and the sensorimotor cortex of the left hemisphere. To date, such lesions have not been documented in children whose speech production problems have been labeled such names as developmental apraxia of speech or developmental verbal apraxia. This topic will be discussed more thoroughly in later chapters.

Descriptions of apraxia of speech in the adult can be found in Darley, Aronson, and Brown (1975); Johns and LaPointe (1976); and Wertz, LaPointe, and Rosenbek (1984). However, even in the adult population with acquired brain damage, the use of the term *apraxia* to describe a patient's speech problem has been debated (Martin, 1974) and is not unanimously accepted.

Initial use of the term *articulatory dyspraxia* by Morley, Court, and Miller (1954) was perhaps the first suggestion that a specified group of children with articulation problems could best be described with a different term than had previously been used. Interestingly, many of the early articles that addressed a developmental form of apraxia of speech were written by authors who had worked with acquired apraxia of speech of speech. The discussions offered by many of these authors frequently pointed out similarities and differences of symptoms in developmental apraxia of speech and acquired apraxia in adults. Thus, perhaps, the term was borrowed from the adult literature because of its descriptive characteristics. For example, a high incidence of isolated apraxic signs (22/35) was reported in a review Rosenbek and Wertz (1972) made of children, whereas in adults it occurs as a part of a picture of more widespread neurological deficit. Furthermore, phonemic errors, omissions, substitutions, distortions, additions, repetitions, and prolongations may predominate in both acquired and developmental apraxia of speech, though ''unlike the apraxic adult, the child seems to make more sound and syllable omission errors'' (Rosenbek & Wertz, 1972, p. 29). Articulatory inaccuracy is noted to increase with response length for both developmental and acquired apraxia of speech. Our clinical experiences suggest that the most important similarity that exists between the groups, and between individuals within the groups, is the lack of volitional control of the oral mechanism for speech production. The similarities or differences between the overt symptoms in the adults with acquired apraxia and the child with DAS may be entirely due to the nature of apraxia and may also be a function of its occurrence in relationship to the child's stage of speech development.

In spite of similarities observed between the speech behaviors of children with developmental apraxia of speech and adults with acquired apraxia of speech, the fact remains that a neurological basis has not been convincingly demonstrated in the children. Although we use a more restricted definition of the term developmental apraxia of speech than Aram (1984) uses for "developmental verbal apraxia," we concur with her hope that use of the term apraxia is not misleading by implying a neurological basis where none has been demonstrated (Rosenbek & Wertz, 1972; Ferry et al., 1975; Aram & Glasson, 1979; Horwitz, 1984). Nevertheless, we do recognize that for many authors "the assumption is made that the problem is due to a neurological impairment" (Bernthal & Bankson, 1988, p. 175). We do not make such an assumption and our statements are not intended to imply the existence of neurological impairment in this population. At the present time, it may be that tools for measuring neurological behaviors are not sensitive or sophisticated enough to detect the critical differences that may exist in this population. In spite of this and other criticisms of the diagnosis of DAS, we do believe that the population exists.

Distinguishing Developmental Apraxia of Speech From Other Childhood Speech Disorders

A common complaint about the use of the term developmental apraxia of speech is that ". . . the vague characterization of developmental apraxia of speech makes it impossible to distinguish from other childhood speech disorders" (Guyette & Diedrich, 1981, p. 8). Studies by individuals attempting to define apraxia of speech in children have frequently described or measured a variety of characteristics of a group of children in an attempt to delineate the feature, or cluster of features, that would permit clinicians to distinguish developmental apraxia of speech from other communication disorders. To date, no effort has been successful. We attribute many of the failures to the makeup of the subject groups. Consider the following subject group of 12 children:

three children with expressive language problems and apraxia,

four children with delayed language development and apraxia,

two children with "soft signs" of neurological involvement and apraxia

two children with mental retardation and apraxia

one child with oral sensory-perceptual deficit and apraxia

An attempt to look for a common profile will undoubtedly meet with failure if the children are evaluated with tools sensitive to language development, syntax, an intelligence test, an oral form discrimination task, and a neurological examination. Using these tools, the common feature of the group—apraxia—is not addressed. As illustrated by the preceding subject group, only evaluation of speech production addresses the common feature of such children. One must take care to control for age and history of remediation. Then, we believe, we will be sensitized to the key features of the disorder of developmental apraxia of speech. This is not to suggest that language development, expressive language problems, or intelligence levels should be ignored. However, they should be recognized along with apraxia of speech as co-occurring problems with no assumption that they represent different aspects of a single syndrome.

We believe that the term developmental apraxia of speech should be used to define the behavior at the locus of our concern—speech. It is our opinion that children may exhibit developmental apraxia of speech as a component of a variety of symptom clusters, but that the use of the term itself should make no implications about any aspect of motor acts, speech, or language other than production of purposeful speech movements. That is, when making this diagnosis, we focus on speech production and the performance of the speech mechanism during speech acts.

Of course, a thorough diagnostic battery must include evaluation of all aspects of a child's communication status. Although other deficits in performance may be revealed, we do not automatically assume that they are a feature of the developmental apraxia of speech. Nevertheless, they need to be considered in the diagnostic procedure and in planning appropriate remediation. The course of development of the child's skills in one area of deficit or strength needs to be considered in light of the restrictions imposed by other deficits or strengths and vice versa. The consequences of one disorder on the performance of other behaviors need to be recognized. This is the role of differential diagnosis and appraisal. It is our contention that such an approach allows for the most efficacious approach to diagnosis and remediation for the child with developmental apraxia of speech.

Developmental Apraxia of Speech: Two Views

Perhaps a review of various ways to look at the interaction of articulation problems and language in children will clarify the strength that resides in separating these behaviors when using the diagnosis of apraxia. One view sees language and articulation as a single entity. Much of the research to date reinforces the idea that the speech and language components of a child's communication disorder are inseparable. Some of the terms used for disorders which encompass apraxia of speech (even developmental apraxia of speech), are used to imply that apraxia, language deficits, and learning disabilities exist as one syndrome.

The single-entity view can be found throughout the literature dealing with apraxia in children. Greene (1967), discussing "articulatory dyspraxia," reported that there was "always an accompanying language disorder" (p. 140). In one of her earlier papers, Aram and Glasson (1979) reported that "developmental apraxia of speech is not confined to the articulatory or motor aspects of speech" (p. 15). In later papers, (1980, 1982) Aram adopted the term *"developmental verbal apraxia"* because it "denotes that the expressive disorder is not confined to speech, but includes all other aspects of verbal expression" (1980, p. 2), and she noted that she viewed developmental verbal apraxia as a "language and articulatory disorder" (1982, p. 2). Crary (1982) referred to *"developmental verbal dyspraxia"* as a term used to describe children presenting "expressive language disorders encompassing both phonology and syntax" (p. 2). Ekelman and Aram (1983, 1984), in studies of spoken syntax in children with "developmental verbal apraxia," reported that their findings "suggest that in addition to motor, speech, or phonological problems, verbally apraxic children also present syntactic disorders in their spoken language" (1983, p. 108). Crary, Landess, and Towne (1984) report that an analysis of phonological error patterns in a group of children with symptoms consistent with Developmental Verbal Dyspraxia "confirms the observations that this clinical entity is an 'expressive' linguistic disturbance. . . . The linguistic problems described may be related to underlying sensory motor deficits responsible for limitations and motor planning" (p. 169).

Such an approach to conceptualizing the communication disorder of these children bundles all system clusters into a single syndrome. We believe that this is a disadvantage to the child because it implies that all behaviors are accounted for or explained. Moreover, it impacts upon the type of remediation program developed for, and used with, the child.

A second view of the relationship between DAS and language is held by a group of authors who discuss developmental apraxia of speech and separate the apraxic features from other behaviors that may accompany it. Morley, Court, and Miller (1954) state "the condition may or may not be associated with delayed development of language" (p. 10). Air and Wood (1985) report "children diagnosed as presenting apraxia of speech often demonstrate other associated problems" (p. 279). In her discussions of symptoms and treatment of developmental apraxia of speech, Haynes (1985) states that "delay in the development of either speech or language is not inherent as a sequela of the disorder" (p. 261). Rosenbek and Wertz (1972) studied 50 children diagnosed with apraxia of speech by a speech pathologist and a consulting neurologist. They note that only 9 of their 50 apraxic children had isolated apraxia of speech. Their observations are consistent with our belief that the diagnosis of DAS should be based on the child's speech production and the performance of the speech mechanism during attempts at speech production. Other behaviors, though they may co-occur, are not a part of DAS.

Still another approach to the definition of the problem demonstrates how subject selection can color our view of the relationship between language and DAS. With the intention of identifying behaviors "which might distinguish developmental apraxia of speech from 'functional' articulation disorders," Yoss and Darley (1974) selected 30 children they considered to be potential candidates. All of their subjects had "normal intelligence, hearing, and language abilities." Although questions may be raised about the test selected to assure "normal language development," their intention is clear: to identify behaviors in a group of apraxic children who had normal language development. The work of Yoss and Darley has become identified as one of the first efforts to systematically document the characteristics of developmental apraxia of speech. The fact that their subjects did not demonstrate a language delay is often cited; the observation that their subject selection criteria excluded language-delayed children is often omitted.

Developmental Apraxia of Speech: As the Authors See It

In summary, developmental apraxia of speech does not refer to a syndrome but designates the locus of our concern—speech. DAS may consist of a variety of symptoms, as we will discuss. This makes it a difficult diagnosis to make—or to discuss—because we believe no one symptom must be present to warrant this diagnosis. We focus on speech production and the performance of the speech mechanism in making the diagnosis.

It may be of historical interest to the clinician to review highlights of developmental apraxia of speech that are consistent with this philosophy. The first case study to appear in the literature was written in 1891 by W.B. Hadden, a British physician. His presentation of "Charles M." described a speech production pattern that was similar to *aphemia,* the term for acquired adult apraxia of speech used in that period. Hadden's description of the eleven-year-old is quite consistent with descriptions presented today when discussing developmental apraxia of speech.

Sixty years later, Morley, Court, and Miller (1954) used the term *articulatory dyspraxia* "to draw attention to a group of children in whom dysarthria is unassociated with any neuromuscular abnormality elsewhere" (p. 10). Morley, Court, Miller, and Garside (1955) ascribe *articulatory apraxia* as a cause of delayed speech. In the first edition of text *The Development and Disorders of Speech in Childhood,* Morley (1957) provided lengthy descriptions of twelve children with developmental articulatory apraxia as well as suggestions for treatment for *articulatory dyspraxia*. In 1969, Morley and Fox furthered the contribution of the British speech-language pathology literature to the history of developmental apraxia of speech through an article that expanded on the theory and suggested remedial goals and procedures for apraxic children.

In the United States, Johnson and Myklebust (1967) discussed *verbal apraxia* within the confines of auditory expressive language disorders. Their text, Learning Disabilities: Educational Principles and Practices, includes a brief description of the disorder, as well as educational procedures to "teach . . . control of the oral musculature" (p. 125). An explosion of interest in this topic is reflected in American journals during the 1970s initiated by Rosenbek and Wertz (1972) who described 50 children they thought warranted the diagnosis of DAS. The first published study to look at the disorder empirically, followed (Yoss & Darley, 1974a). Later the same year two papers dealing with remediation of DAS were published by Rosenbek, Hansen, Baughman, and Lemme (1974) and Yoss and Darley (1974b). Since the mid-1970s the increase in the number of convention papers and other contributions to the literature reflects the growth of interest in the disorder area.

Our goal in writing this book is to attempt to provide a definition of developmental apraxia of speech that will be useful in clarifying the common features addressed by clinicians and in research regardless of how the authors view the other symptom clusters in which it resides. Based on our experiences attempting to locate research subjects, we do not believe that it is a common disorder.

We view DAS as a disorder of motor control of speech production, not attributable to other problems of muscular control. This becomes obvious as the discrepancy between the child's volitional control of the oral mechanism for speech production and that of his peers becomes increasingly noticeable. This book, then, reflects our current state of sophistication with regard to definition, description, and remediation of the disorder. It is our most sincere wish that the readers will approach the ideas thoughtfully, test them, discard them where they prove to be false, expand them where they prove to be inadequate, and use them when possible to help the children who lack verbal control over their world as a result of developmental apraxia of speech.

CHAPTER 2

Speech Characteristics of Developmental Apraxia of Speech

Methodological Problems

Clinically, a central issue in the discussion of DAS is the actual speech characteristics the children exhibit in their attempts at oral communication. There is much information in the literature concerning the speech characteristics of the disorder. However, the literature includes inconsistencies and contradictions. Careful reading suggests that methodological issues may be responsible for the differences, to date, in descriptions of DAS speech characteristics. These problem areas need to be addressed to better understand the present body of DAS literature.

One difficulty encountered when attempting to interpret the DAS literature is the actual format in which the information is reported. Much information is contained in published case studies, clinical reports, and observations, but while these are valuable, perhaps they were obtained and reported with less rigor than if they had been studied systematically. Empirically obtained information demonstrates this needed rigor yet presents problems of a different nature. In such studies the speech characteristics of an individual child may be obscured because of the selection of statistical procedures which emphasize the central tendencies, or the average performances, in a data set generated from a group of DAS subjects.

Another problem with the methods used in studies found in the existing literature is the lack of uniform criteria used for subject selection or inclusion. Subjects of varying ages, intellectual levels, language abilities, and severity of problems are present within the studied subject groups. This complicates comparisons of results across studies. In other reports and studies subject descriptions are absent, which also complicates or invalidates cross-study comparisons.

An additional problem when one tries to describe the speech of children with DAS is that the characteristics on which such a diagnosis is made are seldom thought to be uniquely descriptive of DAS. Many of the

9

same characteristics may also be recognized as exhibited by children with functional/phonological speech sound disorders. However, we think that the clustering of a number of speech characteristics makes possible the DAS diagnosis.

We will now explore the speech characteristics, as described in the present body of literature, which may be evident in individual members of the DAS population. We will also provide suggestions to assist clinicians in assessing these speech characteristics. In this, and the remaining chapters, there will be numerous labels (e.g., *developmental verbal dysphagic, motor aphasic, phonologic programming syndrome,* etc.) which we have highlighted, because we believe the terms refer to similar children that we diagnose as exhibiting DAS.

Speech Sound Errors

The literature contains descriptions of many different types of speech errors being produced by children exhibiting DAS. Although the speech of any single child with DAS could contain a number of different types of errors, for the purposes of this chapter we will now attempt to categorize and describe these errors.

Errors in Sound Class and Manner of Production

Phoneme acquisition has been found to have a general developmental pattern in normal children (Roe & Milisen, 1942; Templin, 1957). Therefore, any discussion of research dealing with deviations of sound class and manner of production must be considered within the framework of the chronological and mental ages of the subjects involved in the study.

Rosenbek and Wertz (1972) found that the 50 children they studied erred most frequently on fricatives, affricates, and consonant clusters. Because this was a retrospective study of data collected by file review, no standard protocol was used to obtain the speech information. At least three different speech-language pathologists had completed the testing. No overt "calibration" of transcription skills specifically for research purposes was reported to have occurred among the examiners. No information regarding severity of the problem or intelligence of the subject group was provided. Because of the wide age range (2 years, 9 months to 14 years) it is difficult to attribute meaning to these findings.

Crary (1984b) reviewed a series of studies focusing on speech sound characteristics of *developmental verbal dyspraxia* (DVD) with which he had been involved. All DVD subjects for each of the studies met the same criteria for inclusion, which were: normal receptive language skills, significant deficits in expressive language skills, normal hearing, no evidence of "intellectual difficulty," no evidence of motor weakness, and demonstrated multiple articulation errors. Crary reported most errors were made in the sound classes involving the more complex oral gestures. Subjects made the most errors on clusters, followed by fricatives, affricates, stops, and nasals. Considering the average age of most of the four subject groups: 7 years, 5 months; 7 years, 4 months; 4 years, 10 months; and 12 years, 8 months, these results appear to be consistent with the general acquisition of sound classes described in normal children.

Dissatisfaction with the cross-sectional nature of many of the studies in the literature prompted Jackson and Hall (1987) to conduct a retrospective longitudinal study of the changes occurring in the speech of four individual children exhibiting DAS. Variability in the children's performances across the years was noted, but individual trends were present within their error patterns. For example, Subject SV was studied from 3 years, 1 month, to 5 years, 3 months of age. During this time period errors in stops and nasals, present when first tested, reduced in number during the second year and were no longer present during the final evaluation. Errors in later learned sound classes, such as fricatives, affricates, liquids, glides, and vocalics, also reduced in number over the time period studied. At the age of 5 years, 3 months, errors occurred only with fricatives and affricates.

Subject PO in the Jackson and Hall study was judged to be more severely disordered than Subject SV, and this was reflected in the longitudinal data as well. He was followed from 4 years, 4 months to the age of 10 years, 7 months. During early evaluations conducted at our clinic PO exhibited problems with production of nasal phonemes. The evaluation conducted when he was 6 years, 7 months suggested resolution of these errors. He gradually reduced the percent of errors on stop productions until he was 7½ years of age. While fricative, affricate, liquid, and vocalic errors decreased over the years studied, some errors continued to be present during the last assessment conducted at age 10 years, 7 months.

We have discussed two of the subjects in the Jackson and Hall longitudinal study in some detail because these children are well-known to us. As was found in previous cross-sectional studies, fricatives and affricates were the most consistently misarticulated phonemes. The data, to date, indicate that the pattern generally seen as normal children develop classes of speech sounds is also present in the children with DAS. However, the Jackson and Hall longitudinal study illustrated that the apraxic children may be acquiring these sounds at a much slower rate, at older ages, and possibly only with the assistance of fairly intensive remedial services.

Unusual Errors

Studies looking closely at the speech production of children with DAS report types of errors typically not seen in the productions of children with speech sound disorders.

ADDITION ERRORS.   Children with DAS may make speech more complicated for themselves by producing extra phonemes in their speech attempts. Such errors were reported by Rosenbek and Wertz (1972) and Yoss and Darley (1974a). The latter authors noted that addition errors occurred in both repetition tasks and in spontaneous speech tasks. They also noted that another type of addition error, that of syllable addition, occurred during production of polysyllabic words. We also have frequently noted the presence of addition errors in the speech of children with DAS seen in our clinic. Examples transcribed from the utterances of children with DAS include the following:

/æpl̩ saks/ for applesauce

/kəloud/ for cloud

/kwink/ for queen

/jʌnjɪnz/ for onions

/klæt/ for cat

/sutskeɪs/ for suitcase

/spreɪs/ for space

The intrusive schwa during cluster production (epenthesis) seems to be a frequent addition error made by children exhibiting DAS. While many children with functional articulation disorders also commit this error, particularly during intervention focused on consonant clusters/blends, the children with DAS seem to make the error more frequently and find it more difficult to eliminate than do children with functional disorders.

PROLONGATION ERRORS.   Rosenbek and Wertz (1972) and Yoss and Darley (1974a) noted the occurrence of prolongations in the speech of their DAS subjects. Yoss and Darley found that this occurred during imitated speech tasks consisting of subject repetition of the investigator's models of consonant-vowel-consonant (CVC), nonsense words, real words, and three syllable words placed in a three-word carrier phrase speech task.

We have also observed this type of error in the speech of the children we have followed with the errors occurring on vowels and continuant consonants. Examples include:

/sːʌn/ for sun

/hæːpi/ for happy

REPETITIONS OF SOUNDS AND SYLLABLES. Rosenbek and Wertz (1972) and Yoss and Darley (1974a) all noted that repetitions of sounds and syllables were present in the DAS speech samples they reported. Yoss and Darley noted this to occur in the context of imitated speech tasks. Aram and Glasson (1979), as reported in Aram and Nation (1982), also noted "trial and error groping kinds of repetitions" (p. 152). In a later section of this chapter we will address repetition errors in relation to disfluency.

Examples of such repetitions noted in the speech transcriptions of our clients exhibiting DAS include:

/s steiɚz/ for stairs

/hæmbɚgɚgɚ/ for hamburger

NONPHONEMIC PRODUCTIONS. Children with DAS occasionally make errors that seem to defy accurate transcription using typical phonetic systems, even when using narrow transcription. Aram and Glasson (1979) noted the presence of glottal plosives and bilabial fricatives. In addition, Yoss and Darley (1974a) cited nasal assimilation and distortions described as subtle voicing and devoicing errors that were not overt substitution errors.

Errors by Type

Speech-language pathologists commonly assess speech patterns by the types of errors produced. Rosenbek and Wertz (1972) reported that their subjects with DAS committed a hierarchy of errors with omission of sounds and syllables being most prominent. These were followed by substitutions, distortions, additions, repetitions, and prolongations—the latter three of which have already been discussed.

Yoss and Darley (1974a) found that different types of errors, related to the complexity of the experimental speech tasks, were committed by subjects whose patterns supported the presence of DAS. For instance, data from imitated speech tasks revealed errors of the following types: two and three feature errors (e.g., /mɪfn/ or /mɪvn/ for *mitten* in which place and/or manner and/or voicing are in error), prolongations and repetitions of sounds or syllables, subtle distortions, and additions. Use of polysyllabic word stimuli resulted in errors of syllable omissions, revisions, and additions. In contrast, when errors from spontaneous speech were analyzed the types of errors committed by the children included distortions, one-place feature errors, additions, and omissions.

Aram and Glasson (1979) divided their subjects into younger and older age groups. Their younger subjects with DAS committed mostly omission and substitution errors. Distortion errors predominated in the older children, who made no unusual substitution errors for single sounds, providing a full phonemic repertoire was present. Aram and Glasson further noted that the older children simplified consonant blends in a variety of ways: via omission of one element, substitution of a less complex phoneme for the entire blend, or production of one correct element while making substitutions for the other element(s).

LaVoi (1986) conducted a cross-sectional study with children presenting DAS. He found that a high percentage of misarticulations consisting of sound omissions was one of three variables which most strongly differentiated the speech of children with DAS from the speech of children with functional articulation disorders.

Jackson and Hall (1987) also addressed type of error in their previously cited longitudinal study of four subjects with DAS. Omission errors occurred most frequently during data collection of the subjects' early years, and as the omission errors decreased, substitution errors either increased or remained at a high level. Substitution errors were the most prevalent type of error for the children over the years studied. Distortion errors were emerging for one of the subjects at the time of their last evaluation on which the study was based. This pattern of error types was also found by Roe and Milisen (1942) in their study of normally developing elementary-school-age children. However, the subjects with DAS were following the pattern at a slower rate than the normal children, thus the correction of error types occurred with them at older ages than with the children developing speech normally.

Voicing Errors

Clinicians frequently report that children with DAS have difficulty producing and maintaining appropriate voicing during their speech attempts. Morley (1959) noted that voiced for unvoiced substitutions were possible errors made by apraxic children. Yoss and Darley (1974a) also noted that voicing errors during imitated speech tasks occurred more than twice as often for the presumed DAS subject group than for a comparative group of articulation disordered subjects. They further noted that subtle voicing and devoicing errors, which Yoss & Darley said could not be called outright sound substitutions, occurred in the speech of the DAS group. Later, Aram and Glasson (1979) reported that voicing errors were variable, with prevocalic voiceless consonants often becoming voiced while final voiced stops became devoiced.

We have found voicing and devoicing errors to be present in the speech of the children with DAS we follow. Such voicing errors were also demonstrated using acoustic analyses of speech samples (Robin, Hall, & Jordan, 1987). This feature, we have found, can be particularly elusive to assess as well as to remediate.

Vowel and Diphthong Errors

Vowels are formed by shaping the oral cavity, whereas consonants are distinguished by constrictions of the oral cavity and can be described by defined contact points. Vowel omissions and misarticulations in the speech of children with DAS have long been clinically observed and reported as demonstrating inconsistencies and variability.

Hadden (1891) listed four vowels and three diphthongs that his patient was unable to "pronounce." It is interesting to note a modification in Morley's views on this topic. In the 1957 edition of her text, she observed that, with the exception of diphthongs in severe cases, vowel and diphthong productions were often normal. Subsequently, in 1959 she noted that vowels and diphthongs could be defective, "the second part of the diphthong being omitted" (p. 97). Misarticulated vowels also have been reported by Rosenbek and Wertz (1972); Lohr (1978); and Davis, Marquardt, and Sussman (1985). On the other hand, Yoss and Darley's (1974a) empirical study did not find vowel errors to be a good variable with which to discriminate between two groups of moderately-to severely-articulation-disordered children, where one group exhibited characteristics consistent with DAS. However, it must be remembered that these conclusions were based on group data, which may have obscured an individual child's performance on speech tasks.

Pollock and Hall (1991) provided individual systematic descriptions of the vowel errors made by five elementary school-age children with severe DAS. The children's spontaneous productions to stimulus objects used in a vowel error screening procedure were recorded and later narrowly transcribed. All the children exhibited errors on rhotic (r and er) vowels and diphthongs, while misarticulations on non-rhotic vowels and diphthongs varied considerably across individual youngsters. However, several common trends were observed. All five children had some difficulty with the tense/lax contrasts (/ɪ/ for /i/, or /i/ for /ɪ/), four of the five had diphthong reduction (/a/ for /aɪ/), and two of the five had difficulty with backing (/a/ for /æ/).

Assessment

The speech of children exhibiting DAS often contains surprises in the form of more unusual or illogical errors than does the speech of children with more predictable speech sound disorders. We find that the axiom of "expect the unexpected" is apropos when inventorying the speech production errors of children with DAS. Therefore, it is incumbent upon clinicians to carefully hone their listening and transcribing skills to accurately record the productions they are assessing.

We find it helpful to assess the articulation skills of children with suspected DAS within a hierarchy of speech tasks. This initially includes an inventory using single words as stimuli. This inventory may be clinician-made or one that is commercially available such as those developed by Pendergast, Dickey, Selmar, and Soder (1969); Templin and Darley (1969); Fisher and Logemann (1971); Compton (1986); Fudala and Reynolds (1986); Goldman and Fristoe (1986); and Hodson (1986). Depending on performance at the single word level of complexity, the clinician may need to reduce the task difficulty level to the isolated phoneme level. Syllable level performance, using a variety of syllable shapes and lengths, such as CV, VC, CVC, C_1VC_2, etc., may also provide useful information. If the child seems able to produce phonemes correctly at the single word level, the clinician can increase the task complexity by introducing multisyllabic words, words placed in different positions of carrier phrases, words in carrier phrases of increasing length, words placed in imitated sentences of increasing length, and by requiring the child to use a target word in an original sentence. Other tasks with greater speech complexity that could be helpful in assessing articulation include observations of, or transcriptions generated from, a reading task or a spontaneous speech sample. However, we caution clinicians to be sensitive to a particular child's reading level before attempting articulation assessment in this context. As will be discussed in Chapter 4, many children with DAS also exhibit learning disabilities.

We have found it helpful to use whole-word transcriptions when analyzing the articulation of children with DAS. Such transcriptions may explain the reasons why particular errors occur. An example from our clinic records was the unusual /l/ for /v/ substitution made during production of the stimulus word *valentine*. The whole-word transcription was /lɛvteɪm/; nestled in an error-riddled production was a metathetic error (discussed later in this chapter) in which the /l/ and /v/ consonants of the first syllable were transposed, thus explaining what initially appeared to be an illogical error.

We urge clinicians to carefully inventory the vowel and diphthong productions of their clients in whom they suspect DAS. Each vowel and diphthong used in the children's regional dialect needs to be assessed across multiple trials and in various phonetic contexts. The placement of stress within the vowel-bearing syllable structure of the word may provide helpful information as well. We have found the vowel error screening procedure described by Pollock and Keiser (1990) to be particularly helpful in this type of assessment which can lead to the development of remedial goals addressing vowel and diphthong errors.

Difficulties Sequencing Phonemes and Syllables

According to the definition of DAS presented in Chapter 1, difficulty in sequencing phonemes is central to the disorder. Problems in correctly sequencing a speech production has been identified by practicing clinicians as a characteristic of DAS (Murdoch, Porter, Younger, & Ozanne, 1984). We define sequencing errors as disruptions in the production of the correct sequencing of phonemes and syllables—the moving from phoneme or syllable A to phoneme or syllable B. The apraxic child may have difficulties in correctly producing phonemes in their appropriate order. An example at the phoneme level could occur, as hereafter described, with production attempts for the /pl/ cluster. An apraxic child who correctly produces the /pl/ cluster in the word *play* is correctly sequencing the phonemes. The addition of the schwa inserted between the elements (/pəl/), the reversal of the consonants (/ləp/), or the omission of one of the cluster's elements are examples of sequencing errors. The substitution of a /w/ for the /l/, or a distortion of the /l/, or the voicing error of /b/ for /p/, are *not* be considered sequencing errors, since movement was accomplished between the two elements of the cluster. Thus sequential movement, itself, is not disrupted.

Hadden (1891) described Charles M., whom we assume exhibited DAS, as having great difficulty "joining consonants and vowels in even simple words" (p. 98). Rapin and Allen (1981) described children with *phonologic programming deficit syndrome* as having difficulties producing speech sounds in correct sequence. Morley (1957, 1965, 1972) noted that some children with DAS may be able to accurately imitate phonemes in isolation but unable to use them in more complex speech tasks or may be able to produce a syllable or isolated word correctly but unable to produce the word in phrases or sentences. Morley (1959) also noted that consonant clusters were more difficult than consonant singles for the child with DAS to produce. McGinnis (1963) described the *motor aphasic* child as having "pronounced difficulties" in sequencing the sounds within words, even though the individual phonemes were within the child's repertoire. Crary (1984b) stated that a major component of the disorder he discussed as *developmental verbal dysphasia* involved production of sound sequences which controlled syllable structure. Chappell (1973) noted sequencing difficulties during the remedial process, stating "sometimes the production of isolated phonemes regressed to an unstable status when the sounds are chained into a sequence" (p. 366).

Results of the study by Yoss and Darley (1974a) found that the group of children with behaviors consistent with DAS had greater difficulty producing multisyllabic words than did their normal controls. That is, the previously discussed omissions, revisions, and additions of syllables affected the syllable integrity of the stimulus words. A study by Williams,

Ingham, and Rosenthal (1981), which replicated the Yoss and Darley design, did not duplicate this finding. However, we speculate that the groups of articulation disordered children studied by Yoss and Darley and Williams, et al. were not, in fact, similar even with a population of children exhibiting severe speech sound disorders. DAS is often thought to be a relatively rare disorder. That is, we question whether the Williams, et al. study had children with DAS within their population of subjects.

Difficulties in sequencing phonemes have also been reported on tasks of speech diadochokinetic rates. Yoss and Darley (1974a) reported that combined syllables, such as /pʌtʌkʌ/, were often produced with syllable sequences in error. This result was also documented in the replication study conducted by Williams, et al. (1981). Aram and Glasson (1979) reported that five of their eight subjects were abnormal in their repetition of the single syllable /pʌ/, and that none of the eight subjects were able to correctly sequence the multisyllabic /pʌtʌkʌ/.

The number of sequencing errors increases as the child encounters greater complexity or length of utterance within the speech task. This was noted by Rosenbek and Wertz in their 1972 review of 50 DAS cases as well as in a report by Ferry, Hall, and Hicks (1975). More recently, Hardcastle, MorganBarry, and Clark (1987) found increased variability within electropalatographic analysis of tongue contacts made during increasingly complex articulatory tasks with two subjects they subsequently diagnosed as exhibiting *verbal dyspraxia*. The two subjects also presented reduced intelligibility in connected speech, as compared with their productions of single words, which the authors believed could be explained by their seeming difficulty with accurate tongue placements in more complex tasks. By contrast, two subjects with speech problems related to dysarthria had less variability in placement than did the two apraxic children.

Metathetic errors are frequently cited in descriptions of DAS. The actual errors result from problems in correctly sequencing sounds and syllables. A child with DAS who transposes or reverses phonemes within a syllable or word, or reverses entire syllables within a word, is committing a metathetic error. Examples include the following transcriptions from clinic notes:

/ʃɪf/ for fish

/mɪsənoda/ for Minnesota

/mæks/ for mask

/ɛfəlʌnt/ for elephant

/soun/ for snow

/hoæmʌá/ for Omaha

/dʒoɚ pak/ for pork chop

These sometimes unusual and occasionally amusing errors are often cited as a characteristic of DAS, although they are errors everyone occasionally makes in the form of Spoonerisms. Morley (1957, 1965, 1972) noted transpositions of sounds and syllables along with the reversals of correct order within the syllables. Johnson and Myklebust (1967) noted a distortion of words as a result of sound transposition. Rosenbek and Wertz (1972) stated that the 50 children exhibiting DAS whose records they reviewed committed frequent metathetic errors. Aram and Nation (1982) also commented on the occurrence of metathetic errors by this population of children.

However, studies by Parsons (1984) and LaVoi (1986), using transcriptions based on administrations of the *Goldman-Fristoe Test of Articulation* (Goldman & Fristoe, 1969), and the *Arizona Articulation Proficiency Scale* (Fudala, 1970), respectively, found that the occurrence of metathetic errors made by children with DAS was not statistically different than the occurrence of such errors made by children diagnosed as having functional articulation disorders. Jackson and Hall (1987) noted the occurrence of metathetic errors in the whole-word transcriptions of two of the four children with DAS included in their longitudinal study. These transcriptions were made from videotaped administrations of the *Templin-Darley Tests of Articulation* (Templin & Darley, 1969). The three articulation assessment tools in the studies cited use numerous monosyllabic words with relatively simple syllable construction. Such stimulus items may have reduced the potential for the occurrence of metathetic errors committed by school-age children. Metathetic errors might have been more evident in these three cited subject populations if more complex speech tasks had been analyzed. It should also be observed that, at least in the Jackson and Hall study, the subjects had received remediation for extensive periods of time, and this factor was believed to have influenced the low incidence of metathetic errors.

Assessment

We have found the breakdown in speech sequencing abilities to be highly individual, dependent upon the severity of the problem and/or the proficiency level the child has achieved. The sequential difficulties in production of consonant singles may be revealed by alteration of the shape of individual syllables. In addition, there may be problems maintaining the correct order of syllables within the production, even if the individual phonemes within each syllable are correctly produced and in the right order. Consonant clusters appear to be particularly troublesome for the child with DAS. Addition errors are observed in the form of intrusive schwas between the cluster elements as well as frequent omission errors of either the entire cluster or some of the cluster's individual component phonemes. Single words consisting of simple syllable shapes may be more easily understood by listeners than the child's attempts at conversational, connected speech simply because of the increased likelihood of more errors occurring in the latter situation.

Assessing a child's ability to sequence speech sounds in a variety of contexts is a crucial element in the diagnostic process and is a valuable use of time by the clinician. Whole-word transcriptions of responses to an articulation assessment instrument will provide rich information on sequencing, especially if it includes a number of consonant cluster target words, as does the *Templin-Darley Tests of Articulation* (Templin & Darley, 1969).

Assessing the agility and control of the oral mechanism for speech production may be particularly helpful. Tasks of increasing word length may provide information on a child's ability to sequence one, two, and three syllable words (e.g., might, mighty, Mighty Mouse). Whole-word transcriptions allow the clinician to observe whether any phonemes or syllables are added, or deleted, or if they are marked by an inaccurate production. Nonsense utterances of one, two, and three syllables, with a variety of voicing requirements contained from syllable to syllable, may give the clinician a sense of the child's skill levels with utterances of increasingly complex configurations. Replication of the same tasks have helped us document progress over a designated time period.

Metathetic errors can most accurately be identified from whole-word transcriptions. Task complexity appears to influence the occurrence of this type of error. We also question the effect of fatigue on ability to maintain control over sequential speech movements in general. A teenage client with DAS we followed for a number of years reported that she experienced more metathetic errors at the end of a day or when she was tired. Within remedial sessions it is our observation that metathetic errors most often occur when the child confronts a task that is more difficult than others required of them at the time. Though initial productions are correctly produced, metathetic errors also occur during repeated productions of a word.

Inconsistency and Variability of Errors

Inconsistency in speech production has been described in the DAS literature. The reader is cautioned at the outset that the terms *consistency* and *variability* are both found in the DAS literature but are used differently by various authors. When possible, individual author's definitions of the terms are given. This does not mean that we necessarily ascribe to these notions—we give them in order to clearly describe the literature in this area. Further discussions of variability and the relationship to inconsistency will be pursued in Chapter 3.

The initial report of DAS by Hadden (1891) included comments regarding inconsistent speech performance: "He usually pronounced the elementary sounds and letters of the alphabet in the same manner when tested on different occasions. Sometimes, however there were slight variations both in saying them and in repeating the Lord's Prayer . . . in the Lord's Prayer he gave the sound of 'n' and 'm', yet the 'm' and 'n' of his alphabet are both 've'." The report also listed 11 phonemes which the child could produce, but noted that "although existing in his code [they] were not always produced" (p. 97-98).

Over the ensuing century, *inconsistency* was frequently cited as a DAS characteristic and still continues to appear in the current literature (see Table 2.1). Morley (1957) reported that use of speech sounds was erratic, while Johnson and Myklebust (1967) noted that at times apraxic children "forgot" how to produce the sounds they had "learned" during treatment. Rosenbek and Wertz (1972) noted that the errors made by the 50 children they reviewed were highly inconsistent, and the inconsistency seemed related to response complexity. Inconsistency seems to be an important characteristic that practicing clinicians use in identifying children with possible DAS. This was verified by Murdoch, et al. (1984), who found that inconsistency was one of the characteristics identified by Australian speech-language pathologists as a diagnostically significant feature of the disorder.

None of the previously cited authors in this section provided operational definitions for inconsistency and variability. Schumacher, McNeil, Vetter, and Yoder (1986) used Mlcoch and Square's (1984) definitions of the terms consistency and variability. They defined consistency as the tendency to misarticulate the same words over repeated trials, while variability was defined as the tendency to produce different errors within the same word and word positions during repeated trials. Both consistency and variability were examined in the speech errors made by three subject groups: children exhibiting normal articulation, children exhibiting functionally disordered articulation, and children exhibiting DAS. The subjects with DAS were found to misarticulate the same words in repeated trials (consistency), and to produce different errors when the words were repeated (variability). By contrast, the children exhibiting functional articulation problems were consistent, but not variable. This particular study is of importance because it is one of the few providing data that contrasts children with DAS and children with functional articulation problems.

Weiss, Gordon, and Lillywhite, in their 1987 textbook on articulatory and phonologic disorders, also address and define inconsistency and variability in a section devoted to the symptoms of *verbal dyspraxia*.

Inconsistency was defined as "the correct and incorrect productions of the same phonemes within the same word or utterances," and variability was described as the situation in which a "phoneme is produced differently from one time to the next" (pp. 259–260).

The definition of variability used by Weiss et al. addresses an additional area of clinical concern: the comparison of errors over time. Will the child with DAS produce the same errors in a word on Wednesday as were produced in that word on Monday? On two separate days, Betsworth and Hall (1989) videotaped a group of children with DAS producing the stimulus words contained on the *Compton-Hutton Phonological Assessment* (Compton & Hutton, 1978). The analysis indicated that variability in errors was present between the first and second administrations of the test. The subjects produced different errors within the same speech units over repeated trials, with 60% to 86% of the stimulus words showing evidence of this variability.

However, as Aram and Nation (1982) note, there are discrepancies existing in the literature regarding the presence or absence of inconsistencies and variability within the speech of children exhibiting DAS. Edwards (1973) noted that a lack of consistency seemed to be involved in DAS, but was the first to state that there was usually some overall systematic pattern within these errors. Bowman, Parsons, and Morris (1984) postulated that the inconsistent errors reported in the literature may actually have been ruled based, and that consistency itself might have been found if the co-occurring phonologic contexts, situation contexts, nature of the tasks, and learning effects also had been examined. The seven DAS subjects participating in their study performed six speech tasks ranging in difficulty from a spontaneous contextual speech sample to imitation of examiner-modeled single words. No task involved multiple trials. All protocols underwent analysis for 24 phonological processes. The mean rankings of the processes revealed that cluster reduction was the most frequently used process, followed by liquid simplification, stopping, glottal replacement, final consonant deletion, fronting, devoicing, epenthesis, and prevocalic voicing. The investigators reached three conclusions: (a) inconsistency may be an artifact of the manner in which the errors are investigated, (b) inconsistency in use of phonological processes does not seem to be a characteristic of DAS, and (c) children with DAS use consistent types and frequencies of phonological processes between various linguistic tasks and performance loads. Parsons (1984), when comparing the actual processes used by the Bowman et al. (1984) subjects, concluded that the children with DAS used more multiple processes than the non-DAS group and suggested that multiple processes might lead a listener to believe error inconsistency was present.

The conclusion that the speech sound errors made by children presenting DAS are rule-oriented has been reached by investigators who have used a phonological-processes approach to the study of speech sound errors. This orientation also regards phonology as a component of the child's language system with the speech problems themselves being problems of cognitive-linguistic organization. In contrast, and as was discussed in Chapter 1, we regard the articulatory speech problems of children with DAS as a motor-speech disorder, and not one of cognitive-linguistic organization. The studies to date that have used phonological process analyses have not stressed the speech production capabilities with paradigms that would have produced inconsistencies. We postulate that if the subjects in the reviewed studies had been required to repeat the stimuli over additional trials, or on a subsequent day, with a comparison of the actual errors being made, perhaps inconsistencies would have been observed. While the overall processes themselves may have been ranked in a similar order across the additional trials, the individual errors made on the stimuli the processes were based upon could well have been variable. For instance, on trial 1 cluster reduction may be noted on the stimuli *plant, tree,* and *sprinkle,* but on trial 2 these clusters may be correctly produced. However, cluster reduction may be evident during trial 2 on production of other stimuli contained in the assessment test, such as *scratch, bread,* and *glasses.* The unsuppressed processes cited by Bowman et al. (1984) describe errors that we also typically transcribe but describe them using a different orientation to the problem of DAS.

The literature does not present a consensus regarding the consistency or variability of errors committed by children with DAS. Our clinical experiences have lead us to believe that most children with DAS do exhibit some degree of inconsistency within their speech errors, dependent upon the complexity of the task being required of them. Inconsistencies may be particularly apparent when comparisons of the same task over several time periods are made and when repeated trials of the same speech task are required of the children. For instance, the following transcriptions reflect the attempts of one of our clients with DAS to produce the word *refrigerator* three times in immediate succession:

/rɛpɪmɛɚ/

/wɛpɪwæʃɚ/

/hipɪfwæʒɚ/

The same child's productions of "measuring spoons" resulted in the following transcriptions:

/ʌnɛdʒɚ sbun/

/ənɛʃoɚ spun/

/jmɛʃɚ sbʌn/

Errors seem to increase in occurrence and decrease in consistency when the children attempt a new level of task complexity. Use of correct voicing may be particularly problematic for some children with DAS, as is increasing the structural difficulty of the response. We acknowledge that such errors are made by children exhibiting functional or developmental speech sound disorders, as well as those with DAS. In the population of children with DAS, however, it seems as if smaller changes in complexity produce a greater number of errors. Errors become more inconsistent and frequent when the speech system is taxed by increasing the number of repetitions of an utterance the child must produce. By contrast, children with functional articulation disorders may actually improve their productions with the increased practice multiple trials provide. Finally, with children presenting DAS, inconsistencies may also be apparent in productions separated in time.

Assessment

Assessment for inconsistency and variability involves study of errors across multiple trials and in contexts ranging from imitations to spontaneous speech. Comparison of the same tasks performed on a subsequent day can determine stability of error patterns over time.

We have found repeated speech trials of the same stimuli to be diagnostically helpful. Suggested are speech diadochokinetic tasks for single syllables, bisyllables, and trisyllables. These stimuli have been developed to address the consistency of performance issue. For those children who do not demonstrate a breakdown within three repetitions, in order to stress the system the authors suggest pursuing each task over at least five trials. Bisyllable stimuli could be designed to provide a variety of voicing combinations that may make it possible to assess for consistency of productions across trials. It is suggested that the examiner make on-line transcriptions of the consonants for each trial as they are being produced.

Tasks involving increasing word length provide information about consistency of errors as the complexity of syllable number increases. Clinicians may need to be selective about which words are presented to any particular client so that no phoneme is overly represented within the stimuli.

Another task involving production of multisyllabic words across multiple trials may also provide helpful information about the consistency of phoneme production using a variety of stress patterns. We use stimulus words that increase from two to five syllables in length. Included are some four-syllable and five-syllable stimulus words containing a weak syllable (*macaroni* and *Tyrannasaurus*). We suggest that the words be produced across a minimum of three trials. Of course, additional trials may provide insight about the child who seems to have little, or minimal, difficulty with the suggested three trials. Comparisons of performance on the longer words that do, and do not, contain the weak syllables also may be helpful in assessing production consistency. Additionally, we find the multisyllabic words and stimulus pictures from the *Assessment of Phonological Processes–Revised* (Hodson, 1986) helpful materials when produced across a number of trials. These assessment tasks may also be helpful in determining stability of errors over time.

Although designed to help with the diagnostic description of the speech skills in DAS, clinicians may also find the above listed types of tasks helpful in assessing stability of speech skills as remediation progresses. Further, the goal of consistency of productions should become an important component of remediation and not remain solely a diagnostic issue. Clinicians can assess consistency or stability of speech production and inconsistency of errors by the careful gathering and analysis of performance data collected on target phonemes during remedial sessions. We suggest that clinicians be alert to errors the child makes on non-target phonemes as well. Our impression from such data is that the performance and progress of children demonstrating DAS is often unpredictable due to the child's inconsistency. In addition, performance may vary as speech task levels change within the remedial context. Such observations made within the remediation setting can become very important when assessing whether inconsistency is an aspect of the speech of children with DAS and in the description of it. Our experience has been that performances of children with DAS are variable and inconsistent both within and between sessions. Therefore, the clinicians who have constant contact with the child may ultimately provide the most pertinent information about any one individual child's consistency of performance based on information obtained over long time frames.

Intelligibility

The intelligibility of DAS children's speech has also been addressed in the literature. Hadden (1891) described his patient's speech as being "quite unintelligible. . . . .even the simplest words, such as 'cat,' could not be rendered so as to be recognized by others." The patient's sister was reported to be the only one who "professed" to understand his speech, although Hadden questioned if she could understand the "details," even when she was able to "make out what he meant" (p. 97). Rosenbek and Wertz (1972) stated in their review of 50 children with DAS that "connected speech was more unintelligible than would be expected on the basis of single-word articulation test results." Edwards (1973) noted a similar pattern when she wrote that "imitation of single words and of short automatic phrases may be reasonable, but stretches of spontaneous creative speech may be unintelligible." Lohr (1978) said that many words used in the expressive language attempts of children with DAS were unintelligible. Aram and Glasson's (1979) descriptions of older children exhibiting developmental verbal apraxia, cited by Aram and Nation (1982), noted variability in speech intelligibility, which was dependent upon the length and complexity of the utterances. The least intelligible context was conversational speech. This coincides with our observation that children with DAS are the most unintelligible in conversational speech, particularly when the listeners lack knowledge of the topic or context. Perhaps the lack of reinforcement from listeners drives children with DAS to hesitate to enter speaking situations and thereby results in less experience with novel speaking activities and variable practice.

Assessment

Speech intelligibility may be closely related to the severity of the problem. Although attempts have been, and are being made, to objectify measures of intelligibility (e.g., Yorkston & Beukelman, 1984; and Monson, Moog & Geers, 1988), ratings of speech intelligibility are generally based on subjective elements within the diagnostic process. Because to many it addresses the reason for remediation, ratings of speech intelligibility are a valuable aspect of assessment as long as the parameters upon which they are based are well described.

The complexity level of the speech tasks needs to be considered. For instance, particularly with the child exhibiting DAS, as the speech task becomes more difficult, intelligibility is likely to decrease. Thus a child may be intelligible in CVC words, but when these same words are placed in a connected speech situation, they may become unintelligible because of increased errors in the CVC. Even if the CVC word is correctly produced in connected speech, the other words produced in the utterance may be unintelligible so that the intended message is not successfully produced.

The listener's knowledge of the topic is a factor that must also be considered. If a topic is known, there is an inherent limiting of the words that are likely to be attempted. This increases the predictability of the words being used, as well as the probability of the listener "understanding" the words used, even from partial cues, if the words are not produced totally correctly.

The listener's familiarity with the speech of the child with DAS is another parameter that must be considered when evaluating intelligibility. Individuals who frequently interact with the child may be able to decode utterances that are unintelligible to others. Perhaps this is because frequent associations with the child help a person identify consistencies that may exist within the speech patterns. Frequent associations also allow the person to know the child well enough to predict what topics are likely to be discussed and to be familiar with details about the child's life. This allows the listener to "fill in" or correct words or utterances that are deviant in the child's actual oral productions.

Yet another factor that may affect intelligibility is the presence or absence of nonverbal cues. If the listener is restricted to only auditory cues, the DAS child's intelligibility may be evaluated as poorer than when the listener is interacting directly with the youngster. Therefore, audio-taped evaluations of intelligibility may result in different ratings than when visual cues are also available. This may be one reason why a listener may find it far more difficult to converse over the telephone with a child exhib-iting DAS where no visual cues are available than in chatting with the child face to face. Direct interactions allow the listener to benefit from visual cues, receiving not only information from the oral attempts at com-munication but also from the child's facial cues, gestures, and general body language. These added visual cues may increase the ease with which the listener understands the child, thus elevating the subjective rating of the child's intelligibility.

The degree of training individual listeners have with disordered com-munication will affect skills in making subjective evaluations of intelligi-bility for many of the reasons previously discussed. A speech-language pathologist may be able better to compensate for the speech production problems of the child with DAS than a novice because of the speech-language professional's training and experience in dealing with disordered communication.

Thus, in rating the speech intelligibility of a child with DAS, the clini-cian will need to recognize and describe multiple factors. These include the context in which the judgment was made, the complexity of the speech task or tasks on which the judgment(s) are made, the listener's familiarity with the topic, and the listener's familiarity with the individual child's speech patterns.

Severity of the Problem

Many authors (see Table 2.1) have stated that children with DAS exhibit severe speech disorders or imply this in their case reports. The inclusion of "severe" as a descriptor of the problem may be a function of the work setting, the clinical bias, and/or research methodology used by particular authors. For instance, much of the literature has been generated in univer-sity/hospital/clinic environments which are likely to serve as a resource for the more severe problems. If milder cases are not referred, and we suspect they are not, they may be lost to the literature.

In reality, although not readily apparent in the literature, this dis-order presents itself along a continuum of severity. For example, Aram and Nation (1982) state children with *Developmental Verbal Apraxia*

TABLE 2.1

Descriptions or Discussions of Reported Characteristics
of Developmental Apraxia of Speech (DAS)

CHARACTERISTICS	REFERENCES
Errors in sound class and manner of production	Rosenbek & Wertz, 1972 Crary, 1984b Jackson & Hall, 1987
Addition errors	Rosenbek & Wertz, 1972 Yoss & Darley, 1974a
Prolongation errors	Rosenbek & Wertz, 1972 Yoss & Darley, 1974a
Repetition errors	Rosenbek & Wertz, 1972 Yoss & Darley, 1974a Aram & Glasson, 1979
Nonphonemic productions	Yoss & Darley, 1974a Aram & Glasson, 1979
Type of errors	Rosenbek & Wertz, 1972 Yoss & Darley, 1974a Aram & Glasson, 1979 LaVoi, 1986 Jackson & Hall, 1987
Voicing errors	Morley, 1959 Yoss & Darley, 1974a Aram & Glasson, 1979 Robin, Hall, & Jordan, 1987
Vowel and Diphthong Errors	Hadden, 1891 Morley, 1957 Morley, 1959 Rosenbek & Wertz, 1972 Yoss & Darley, 1974a Lohr, 1978 Davis, Marquardt, & Sussman, 1985 Pollock & Hall, 1991 Marquardt & Sussman, 1991

(Continued)

TABLE 2.1 (Continued)

CHARACTERISTICS	REFERENCES
Difficulties sequencing phonemes	Hadden, 1891
	Morley, 1957, 1965, 1972
	Morley, 1959
	McGinnis, 1963
	Eisenson, 1972
	Rosenbek & Wertz, 1972
	Chappell, 1973
	Yoss & Darley, 1974a
	Ferry, Hall, & Hicks, 1975
	Aram & Glasson, 1979
	Rapin & Allen, 1981
	Williams, Ingham, & Rosenthal, 1981
	Crary, 1984b
	Murdoch, Porter, Younger, & Ozanne, 1984
	Hardcastle, MorganBarry, & Clark, 1987
Metathetic errors	Morley, 1957
	Johnson & Myklebust, 1967
	Rosenbek & Wertz, 1972
	Aram & Nation, 1982
	Parsons, 1984
	LaVoi, 1986
	Jackson & Hall, 1987
Inconsistency and/or variability of errors	Hadden, 1891
	Morley, 1957
	Johnson & Myklebust, 1967
	Rosenbek & Wertz, 1972
	Edwards, 1973
	Lohr, 1978
	Aram & Nation, 1982
	Murdoch, Porter, Younger, & Ozanne, 1984
	Bowman, Parsons, & Morris, 1984
	Parsons, 1984
	Schumacher, McNeil, Vetter, & Yoder, 1986
	Weiss, Gordon, & Lillywhite, 1987
	Betsworth & Hall, 1989
	Marquardt & Sussman, 1991

(Continued)

TABLE 2.1 (Continued)

CHARACTERISTICS	REFERENCES
Intelligibility	Hadden, 1891 Rosenbek & Wertz, 1972 Edwards, 1973 Lohr, 1978 Aram & Glasson, 1979 Greene, 1983
Severity of the Problem	Hadden, 1891 Orton, 1937 Morley, 1957 Morley, 1959 Walton, Ellis, & Court, 1962 Court & Harris, 1965 Johnson & Myklebust, 1967 Morley & Fox, 1969 Dabul, 1971 Daly, Cantrell, Cantrell, & Aman, 1972 Eisenson, 1972 Rosenbek, Hansen, Baughman, & Lemme, 1974 Ferry, Hall, & Hicks, 1975 Hunter, 1975 Lohr, 1978 Crary, 1981 Aram & Nation, 1982 Greene, 1983 Sommers, 1983 Crary, 1984a Crary, 1984b Aram, 1984 Harlan, 1984 Love & Fitzgerald, 1984 Deputy, 1984 Perkins, 1984 Hall, 1989 Marquardt & Sussman, 1991

(Continued)

TABLE 2.1 (Continued)

CHARACTERISTICS	REFERENCES
Nasality and/or nasal emissions	Morley, 1957, 1965, 1972 Dabul, 1971 Yoss & Darley, 1974a Aram & Glasson, 1979 Parsons, 1984 Bowman, Parsons, & Morris, 1984 Trost-Cardamone, 1986 Hall, Hardy, & LaVelle, 1990
Groping/silent posturing of articulators	Rosenbek & Wertz, 1972 Chappell, 1973 Yoss & Darley, 1974a Love & Fitzgerald, 1984 Murdoch, Porter, Younger, & Ozanne, 1984 Hall, 1989 Hall, Hardy, & LaVelle, 1990
Prosodic disturbances	Orton, 1937 Morley, 1957 Rosenbek & Wertz, 1972 Edwards, 1973 Ferry, Hall, & Hicks, 1975 Aram & Glasson, 1979 Guyette & Diedrich, 1983 Robin, Hall, & Jordan, 1987 Milloy & Summers, 1989 Hall, 1989 Hall, Hardy, & LaVelle, 1990 Robin, Klouda, & Hug, 1991 Robin, Hall, Jordan, & Gordan, 1991
Fluency	Orton, 1937 Ingram & Reid, 1956 Morley, 1957, 1965, 1972 Aram & Nation, 1982 Milloy & Summers, 1989
Phonologic characteristics	Aram & Glasson, 1979 Crary, 1984b Bowman, Parsons, & Morris, 1984 Parsons, 1984 Jackson & Hall, 1987 Betsworth & Hall, 1989

(Continued)

TABLE 2.1 (Continued)

CHARACTERISTICS	REFERENCES
Prognosis	Orton, 1937
	Morley, Court, & Miller, 1954
	Morley, 1957, 1965, 1972
	Rosenbek, Hansen, Baughman, & Lemme, 1974
	Yoss & Darley, 1974b
	Ferry, Hall, & Hicks, 1975
	Darley & Spriestersbach, 1978
	Macaluso-Haynes, 1978
	Aram, 1980
	Aram & Nation, 1982
	Blakeley, 1983
	Greene, 1983
	Ekelman & Aram, 1984
	Helfrich-Miller, 1984
	Haynes, 1985
	Weiss, Gordon, & Lillywhite, 1987
	Jackson & Hall, 1987
	Air, Wood, & Neils, 1989
	Hall, 1989
	Milloy & Summers, 1989
	Hall, Hardy, & LaVelle, 1990
	Marquardt & Sussman, 1991

"can range from presenting relatively mild disorders to being nonverbal and unable to acquire useful speech" (p. 153). Indeed, Orton (1937) and Morley (1959) report that they have seen children exhibiting DAS with only "lisps" or "defective r's."

A belated recognition of possible "dyspraxic" components in a mild disorder was reported by Love and Fitzgerald (1984). The disorder was recognized after repeated examination of the child and not early in the diagnostic process. Hall (1989) also reported a case study of a child who had a mild problem involving the /r/, /ɜ˞/, and /ə˞/ phonemes. However, as remedial contact with this child continued, Hall became aware of speech behaviors occurring within the child which were consistent with DAS, including inconsistency of performance within and between sessions, difficulties producing multisyllabic words, as well as groping of the oral mechanism prior to production attempts. Thus the possibility of DAS was recognized, in a mild form, only after multiple observations of her speech had been made.

Assessment

When diagnosing children with possible DAS, speech-language patholo-gists are urged to be aware that the disorder occurs throughout the sever-ity range of communication disorders. Professionals need to be alert for this possibility even with "mild" speech sound disordered clients as well as with clients who seem to respond poorly to our customary remedia-tion techniques.

Severity ratings of a communication disorder tend to be highly sub-jective and may vary depending upon the clinical experiences of the professional making the judgments. Nonetheless, ratings of severity appear to be an inherent part of all assessments whether made during an actual diagnostic evaluation or as part of on-going contact within a remedial context. Unfortunately, there are few standards of how we actually assess severity; severity may be based on different parameters for different professionals, although attention to a variety of speech characteristics and the estimate of prognosis are probably included. Some clinicians may base this judgment on one observation of articulatory accuracy while others may look at consistency or improvement over a period of time. Still others may address intelligibility with little or no control of the listener's knowledge of context. Some clinicians may respond to other unspecified variables.

Our estimates of severity are probably based on a combination of features including, but not restricted to, the child's stimulability, ability to control the environment through use of speech, change over time, degree of developmental lag, and overall intelligibility, as well as the impact of co-occurring problems (to be discussed in Chapters 4, 5, and 6).

Nasality/Nasal Emission

Parents, teachers, or clinicians of children with suspected DAS who are referred to the University of Iowa's Wendell Johnson Speech and Hearing Clinic sometimes complain of "nasal voice quality." Morley (1957, 1965, 1972) noted that incoordination in use of the nasopharyngeal sphincter could be due to an "articulatory dyspraxia." Dabul (1971) noted a nasal-ized neutral vowel to be the only vocalization initially inventoried in her case study of a 5½-year-old child with apraxia. Associated with the nasal-ized productions was "slow, inefficient function of the velopharyngeal mechanism" (p. 30), although assessment techniques were unspecified. After one semester of remediation, which included no goals directly related to nasal-oral air flow, the child was reported to "better" emit air orally than nasally, but it was also noted that his speech retained a "nasal quality." Yoss and Darley (1974a) noted nasal assimilations in the error patterns of the DAS group of subjects. Aram and Glasson (1979) also noted that some children with apraxia presented assimilation nasality. They further reported that some children also added stops after nasal productions. This type of addition error, described previously in this chapter, has been noted by the authors with the following being transcribed examples:

/kwink/for "queen"
/rɪŋk/for "ring"

Two articles that appeared in 1984 looked at phonological processes, including nasalization and denasalization. Bowman, Parsons, and Morris (1984) ranked 24 processes that occurred in the speech of seven children with DAS across nine different speech tasks. Nasal assimilation ranked fourteenth, denasalization ranked seventeenth, and nasalization ranked nineteenth. In another article dealing with the same seven children, Parsons (1984) found only one of the seven subjects actually exhibited both the denasalization and nasalization processes.

However, we view problems with nasality and denasality in children also presenting other symptoms of DAS as potential evidence of poor motor control of the velopharyngeal mechanism, rather than one of phonological processing. In support of the motor control explanation, Trost-Cardamone (1986) similarly noted that apraxia in children may disturb the speech programming for velopharyngeal port operation, and problems in this programming underlie the oral vs. nasal errors made by some children with DAS. Trost-Cardamone suggests that problems with nasal air flow control may not be prevalent with the majority of children with DAS, but the possibility of the problem needs to be acknowledged.

Hall, Hardy, and LaVelle (1990) followed a child with DAS for 11 years. Among the cluster of symptoms on which the diagnosis of DAS was based was the presence of velopharyngeal dysfunction resulting in inappropriate nasal resonance and nasal emission. When initially evaluated at the age of 7 years, the child's significant hypernasality and increased nasal emission within more complex speech contexts was thought to contribute to her lack of intelligibility. Her velum was asymmetrical at rest and during phonation. Nasal airflow rates revealed that the velopharyngeal incompetence resulted from the mechanism not accomplishing appropriate speech production gestures, rather than from a specific palatal disability such as paralysis or structural abnormalities. Palatal management was initially deferred to determine whether intensive articulation remediation affected velopharyngeal function. Following 6 weeks of intensive intervention, inappropriate nasal airflow continued to be present during speech attempts. However, the client also produced some phonemes correctly where there was little or no nasal airflow indicating that occasional velopharyngeal closure or minimal openings had occurred, even though the port was inappropriately open during the majority of speech attempts. This same pattern continued to be present after a second 6 week period of intensive remediation at which time a palatal lift prosthesis was constructed. (See Figures 2.1 and 2.2.)

With the compensation for velopharyngeal closure, the client was able to impound intraoral air pressures, which facilitated her improving articulation skills. Since the initial construction of the lift, head and jaw growth and atrophy of the adenoidal pad have resulted in several additions being made to the posterior portions of the lift. As well, the lift was modified to accommodate orthodontia. With the lift in place, our client's hypernasality was resolved.

We find that, at some point, most children exhibiting DAS have problems with hypernasality, hyponasality, or nasal emissions. Sometimes this is quite subtle, in most instances, it is variable and inconsistent in occurrence. This observation further supports our contention that nasal air flow problems in children with DAS result from problems in motor control and may specifically be related to the timing of velar movement.

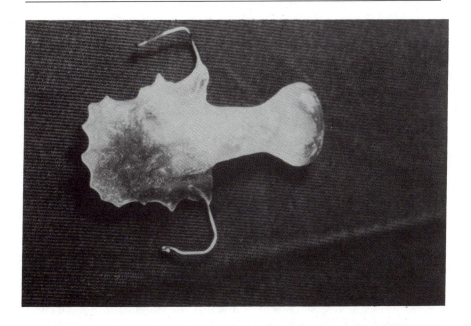

FIGURE 2.1. Palatal lift prosthesis. *Note.* From ''A child with signs of developmental apraxia of speech with whom a palatal lift prosthesis was used to manage palatal dysfunction'' by P. K. Hall, J. C. Hardy, & W. E. LaVelle, 1990, *Journal of Speech and Hearing Disorders, 55,* 454–460. Reprinted by permission.

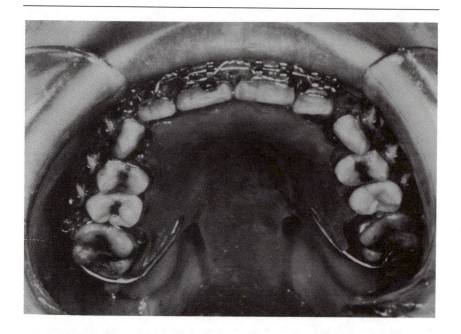

FIGURE 2.2. Palatal lift prosthesis in place (anterior portions are modified to accommodate orthodontia). *Note.* From "A child with signs of developmental apraxia of speech with whom a palatal lift prosthesis was used to manage palatal dysfunction" by P. K. Hall, J. C. Hardy, & W. E. LaVelle, 1990, *Journal of Speech and Hearing Disorders, 55,* 454–460. Reprinted by permission.

Further, our experience has been that many children with DAS exhibit asymmetrical palates with uvular deviations at rest and during phonation of /a/, which may indicate potential palatal management problems. We perceive a high incidence of nasality in our population of DAS clients which is probably related to our association with an effective palatal lift team (LaVelle & Hardy, 1979) and which has sensitized us to carefully evaluate the velopharyngeal function in these children.

The velopharyngeal mechanism must be considered an integral part of the speech mechanism. When DAS is present, this mechanism could well exhibit dysfunction, just as do the lips and tongue, during the complex sequential movements that must be achieved during speech production. In addition, velopharyngeal port problems create difficulty in impounding the intraoral air pressures needed to produce most American English consonants, thus further complicating the speech production tasks of the child with DAS.

Assessment

The diagnosis of hypernasality and hyponasality requires a subjective judgment. This may depend somewhat on regional speech variations and the degree to which nasality is acceptable. Overt nasal emissions require careful monitoring on the part of the clinician. Nares flaring during productions of stops and sibilants could signal such emission. Another technique helpful in assessing the presence or absence of appropriate nasal air flow is the use of a ''nasal mirror.'' A small mirror can be placed under the child's nares during speech, with clouding on the surface occurring when nasal air is emitted. The clinician must then determine if the clouding occurred during the production of a nasal, or nonnasal, phoneme.

An examination of the structural and functional adequacy of the speech mechanism is mandatory in the assessment of nasality and velopharyngeal port function. Assessment of structural adequacy, as visually inspected, is needed. Any asymmetry of the structures needs to be noted during rest and during movement. Functional adequacy of the mechanism also needs to be assessed in the form of posterior palatal and mesial lateral wall movements during such tasks as prolonged /a/ and repetitions of /a/.

More elaborate assessments can be made via videofluoroscopy, videoendoscopy, and aerodynamic measures, as well as acoustic measurements of nasality by use of the Nasometer to address problems both of structural adequacy and/or motor control. These may be particularly helpful when questions of adequate palatal length or coordination/timing occur. Of course, some of these procedures are invasive so such assessments should not be routine but reserved for those children about whom there are major questions of functional adequacy of the velum. (For more information on use of these instrumental assessment procedures, please refer to Folkins & Moon, 1990; and Moon, 1993).

Presence of Groping Behaviors or Silent Posturing of Articulators

When asked to describe characteristics of DAS, many practicing clinicians cite the presence of groping and silent posturing of the articulators. This is a rather notable behavior when observed during a child's speech attempts, and a behavior that clinicians are likely to remember. Murdoch, Porter, Younger, and Ozanne (1984), in a survey study dealing with the differential diagnosis of the disorder, found that Australian speech-language pathologists cited this characteristic as one of three that was ''always'' associated with DAS.

Descriptions of DAS in the literature also note the characteristic of groping behaviors and silent posturing (see Table 2.1). Interestingly, in the Yoss and Darley (1974a) study, this behavior was present only in the older subjects, occurring most noticeably during the production of three-syllable words.

While most people in the field refer to groping and silent posturing as a single entity, we believe they are two separate behaviors within the DAS child's attempts to speak. Silent posturing, as we define it, is a static state of articulatory position that occurs without sound production. We define groping as an active and ongoing series of movements of the articulators in an attempt to find the desired articulatory position necessary for correct phoneme production.

Groping and silent posturing are characteristics that may occur with children presenting DAS at some point during our contact with them. Occasionally, apparently out of desperation with their failure to achieve correct articulatory postures, we have observed children with DAS manipulate their articulators with their fingers in an attempt to produce a sound correctly.

Perhaps silent posturing and groping increase after the implementation of remediation when the child's awareness of articulator placement and the child's desire to perform correctly increase. A dependence on such placement feedback in later phases of remediation may encourage the child to practice a gesture prior to its execution. This may explain why Yoss and Darley (1974a) found this behavior only in their older children who were presumably those receiving intervention, and why Hall, Hardy, and LaVelle (1990) report that this feature in the speech behavior of their subject was not noted until she had made some degree of progress within her articulation remediation program. However, we have seen silent posturing occur in preschool children with DAS as well as school age children with the disorder, which may reflect the early identification and service provision of the young preschool population in Iowa.

Assessment

The good observer will profit from attending to the nonverbal behaviors of children with DAS. We find that groping and silent posturing can occur at any point during an evaluation or remedial session. Because of this, we frequently videotape entire evaluation sessions for later review and analysis of a variety of communication skills, including these particular behaviors.

Prosodic Impairment

One characteristic included in many definitions of DAS is a description of abnormal prosody. Prosody refers to variations in three acoustic parameters of the speech waveform (duration, frequency, and amplitude) that may serve to alter the melody of speech and the meaning of spoken language. The communication functions of prosody include conveying emotional tone (Cosmides, 1983; Scherer, 1986; Williams and Stevens, 1972) and linguistic distinctions. The linguistic uses of prosody include stress allocation within an utterance or word (Cooper, Eady, & Mueller, 1985; Selkirk, 1984); the definition of syntactic boundaries (Cooper & Sorensen, 1981), and the difference between interrogative and declarative sentence forms (Eady & Cooper, 1986). Moreover, Wingfield, Lombardi, and Sokol (1984) found that prosody facilitates listeners' determination of syntactic structure and intelligibility.

There have been relatively few reports on prosody usage in children; most studies have been concerned with adults with neurologic lesions (cf. Robin, Klouda, & Hug, 1991). Relatively few studies have documented impaired prosody in subgroups of children with speech and/or language problems. This lack of study is of particular concern in DAS because many investigators and clinicians describe abnormal prosody as one of the features of the disorder.

Statements in the DAS literature about abnormal prosody have been made by Rosenbek and Wertz (1972), Aram and Glasson (1979), Edwards (1973), and Guyette and Diedrich (1983). (Additional references that allude to prosodic difficulties can be found in Table 2.1.) These studies have not examined the prosodic aspect of DAS speech systematically but rather are anecdotal statements about prosodic abilities in children exhibiting DAS.

We have reported on prosodic abilities in children with DAS using perceptual and acoustic measures (Robin, Hall, & Jordan, 1987; Robin, Hall, Jordan, & Gordan, 1991). Robin, Hall, and Jordan (1987) examined the ability of five children with DAS to produce utterances in five different ways: as if they were happy, sad, or angry (emotive conditions) and as a question or as a neutral utterance (linguistic conditions). Both perceptual and acoustic measures of the speech output were then made. When a group of listeners was asked to identify these various utterances produced by the children with DAS, they were accurate only 48% of the time. Most listeners perceived the productions intended to convey emotions (happy, sad, and angry) as "neutral," and the "question" attempts were perceived as happy. The listeners were 80% accurate in identifying the prosodic patterns when they were produced by age and sex matched controls with normal communication skills.

The acoustic data were consistent with the listener's perceptual judgments. However, the acoustic analyses indicated that there was great individual variability between the subjects. Some subjects showed little fundamental frequency distinction between utterances in that the frequency contours were flat. Other children showed variability in fundamental frequency across utterances but did not use the contour appropriately. For instance, sad utterances often had increased variability in the utterance of the DAS subjects while the normal controls showed relatively flat contours. Likewise, the happy utterances were relatively flat with the DAS subjects but were more variable in the normal controls. These differences in fundamental frequency contours were apparent in the speech of the DAS subjects for both the linguistic and the emotive utterances.

Durational analyses of the same data revealed that total sentence durations were longer for the children presenting DAS than the normal control subjects. Most of the children with DAS did not use duration to signal differences in prosodic patterns. However, like the fundamental frequency data, there was intersubject variability. Some of the children with DAS lengthened the final words of sentences for questions (as did the controls), while some did not.

Further analyses revealed that the subjects demonstrating DAS had longer voice onset times (the amount of time between the initial burst of a consonant and the onset of voicing), than did the normal control children for voiced and voiceless sounds. As well, children exhibiting DAS had longer vowel and fricative durations than did the normal control children.

The results of our study confirmed clinicians' impressions that the prosody of children with DAS was, indeed, impaired. However, our results suggest that the disorder manifests itself differently in individual children with DAS. Some of the children could be described as "aprosodic," exhibiting flat prosody or attenuated fundamental frequency variation. Other subjects with DAS could be described as "dysprosodic" in that variations in fundamental frequency and duration were apparent in their speech but not used appropriately.

Robin, Hall, Jordan, and Gordan (1991) also examined the production of sentence focus in children with DAS. In this study, stimuli involved sentences in which one word received focus. Three children exhibiting DAS were studied and their performance compared to three age and sex matched controls. Subjects were tested in their ability to signal stress in a sentence by answering questions designed to place stress on the initial or final word of the sentence or to produce the sentence with a neutral pattern. For example, to elicit stress on the initial word in the sentence, the examiner first made the statement "Dad met Bob" to the children, then asked them to answer the question "Who met Bob?" When asked the question "What happened?," children were told that they were not to stress any word in particular in an effort to elicit a neutral focus. The children were instructed to answer "Who did Bob meet?" in an attempt to elicit stress placement on the final word in the sentence.

As a group, listeners were able to accurately identify the stress productions of the children with DAS 63% of the time, while identification of sentence focus produced by normal children was 81% accurate. Listeners were more accurate at identifying final stress in the sentences produced by children demonstrating DAS but more accurate in the perception of initial stress in utterances of the normal children. Neutral utterances were perceived correctly 38% of the time for the children with DAS and 42% of the time for normal subjects. Thus the children presenting DAS were not only less accurate at producing stress than the normal children, but their pattern of performance was different as well.

Acoustic analyses of the subjects' productions examined peak fundamental frequency for words, word duration, and relative intensity change in words. In our normal subjects, stressed words were usually produced with a higher fundamental frequency and longer duration and were more intense than the same word in a neutral context. However, when the subjects with DAS produced initial words with initial stress or final words with final stress, they produced those words with a lower frequency than they had used in the neutral condition. Eady and Cooper (1986) have noted that normal adult speakers drop fundamental frequency an average of 53 Hz following initial word stress but that this drop is only 23 Hz when the final word is stressed. Our normal control children dropped frequency an average of 53 Hz during initial word stress and 14 Hz when the final word was stressed. By contrast, the children with DAS only dropped fundamental frequency 9 Hz following initial stress and actually increased frequency when the final word was stressed.

Acoustic analyses of word duration and peak intensity level per word were also made. Results were similar to the fundamental frequency findings. For instance, stressed words produced by the subjects exhibiting DAS frequently had lower intensity and shorter duration than unstressed versions of the same word. Normal speakers had the opposite pattern and increased duration and intensity on stressed words. Thus the errors in prosody, perceptually found in children with DAS, correspond to changes in all three parameters of the speech wave form.

Assessment

A complete evaluation of prosodic ability should address both the child's production and perception of intonation. The evaluation should also be structured to obtain information on different aspects of prosody (e.g., emotive uses and linguistic uses). Stimuli should be sentences in which the change in meaning is accomplished by a change in the prosodic contour. Construction of stimuli requires a tape recorder to ensure that each child receives the same utterances on the perception task. Specific emotive patterns to be examined might include happy, sad, and angry. The linguistic distinction between question and neutral should also be examined. The production of stress in a sentence focus task should also be assessed.

Assessment of prosody has been detailed in Robin, Klouda, and Hug (1991). Stimuli for the above as suggested by Robin et al. (1991) are listed in Table 2.2.

Occurrence of Disfluency

Occasional references to disfluencies occurring in the speech of children with DAS have been made. Orton (1937) reported that several children

---

TABLE 2.2
Stimuli Used for Assessment of Prosody

I. Emotive intonation and question and neutral forms
   1. The bird flew away.
   2. Tomorrow I'm leaving for Chicago.
   3. My horse jumped over the fence.
   4. We sold our cottage last month.

II. Emphatic stress
   1. *Don* shot the *puck* to Kent.
   2. *Sheila* took the *money* from *Chip.*
   3. *Stan* paid the *check* for *Peg.*
   4. The *salesperson* sold the *couch* to my *Father.*
   5. *Mary* typed the *paper* for *Kate.*
   6. *Chuck* ate *supper* with *George.*

III. Syntactic juncture sentence pairs
   1. If Harry went to the bank, Ann will be very angry.
      Uncle Harry went to the bank Ann went to yesterday.
   2. If Jerry kicked his mother, we'll be upset.
      If Jerry kicked, his mother will be upset.
   3. Roger went to the concert with Chuck, and Laura went with Rob.
      Roger went to the concert with Chuck and Laura and Rob.
   4. Ellen called Phillip, Bob called Jim, and Sally called Kate.
      Ellen called Phillip, Bob, and Jim, and Sally called Kate.
   5. If the teacher forgot, Jim would remind him.
      If the teacher forgot Jim, we'd remind him.
   6. I went skiing with Jack, and Mike met us there.
      I went skiing with Jack and Mike just last year.
   7. When John left Cindy, we were upset.
      When John left, Cindy was very upset.
   8. If Jimmy used the truck, Sharon will be angry.
      Cousin Jimmy used the truck Sharon used yesterday.

Note. From "Neurogenic disorders of prosody" by Robin, D. A., Klouda, G. V., & Hug, L. N., 1991. In M. P. Cannito & D. Vogel (Eds.), *Treating disordered speech motor control: For clinicians by clinicians* (p. 249). Austin, TX: PRO-ED. Reprinted by permission.

with *developmental motor aphasia* or a *motor speech delay* had stuttered since "beginning to talk;" however, the specific behaviors were not described. Ingram and Reid (1956) noted "irregularities of rhythm" in the speech of 40 *articulatory apraxics* they evaluated. Morley (1957, 1965, 1972) noted that one of her 12 cases had a "stammer" that resolved spontaneously as the articulation improved, while Aram and Nation (1982) noted a disfluent preschool apraxic patient. Also compounding the problem of description is that "repetition" of sounds or syllables has been noted as a DAS error type by Rosenbek and Wertz (1972) and Yoss and Darley (1974a). Unfortunately, descriptions of these disfluencies have not been specific about the kind of behavior that elicited the label. Thus, we do not know whether the behavior is routinely whole word repetition, initial syllable repetition, prolongation of phonemes, or interjections. More careful reporting of observations may delineate specific features that are characteristic of the population with DAS.

Children exhibiting DAS may appear to be disfluent for a variety of reasons. For instance, as we shall explore more fully in a later chapter, children exhibiting DAS often have difficulties with many components of their language skills which may lead to disfluencies of the type described by Hall (1977). The presence of groping and searching behaviors, repetition error types, and disrupted prosodic features may also contribute to disfluent sounding speech. While we have seen many children exhibit these behaviors, we have not yet examined a child in whom stuttering was a co-occurring problem.

Assessment

Differential diagnosis of DAS may be complicated by the appearance of disfluent behaviors. Careful and repeated observation of the child in numerous speech tasks of varying complexities and situations may help determine if disfluent speech behavior is related to DAS or is a separate component needing to be addressed.

Phonologic Characteristics

We view the speech sound production problems of children with DAS as stemming from motor control deficits. However, there is a body of literature addressing this speech disorder from a phonologic-linguistic perspective.

Aram and Glasson (1979) differentiated the phonological characteristics of younger and older children with DAS. They found high vowel to consonant ratios, and simplification errors with the younger children. Aram and Nation (1982) noted that individually, the younger children used a variety of strategies (e.g., reduplications), but these strategies were often used with some degree of regularity. The older children's attempts to produce multisyllabic words contained frequent metathetic errors, syllable omissions, and simplification of blends.

Crary (1984b) analyzed the speech of 20 children with *developmental verbal dyspraxia* and found ten of the 13 studied processes were "strong" in the group since 17 of the subjects exhibited them. All 20 subjects exhibited the processes of final consonant deletion, initial consonant deletion, cluster reduction, and stopping. Errors involving syllable structure simplification were most prevalent. Crary also noted cluster errors were most frequently represented by the reduction of the cluster to a single element.

Parsons (1984) compared seven DAS with seven matched non-DAS phonologically disordered children. The errors in single word utterances were analyzed for the presence of 29 processes, 24 of which were found to actually occur. Cluster reduction and final consonant deletion were the most frequently used processes by both groups. Although the children with DAS demonstrated processes similar to those exhibited by other phonologically impaired children, there were statistically significant differences between the two groups for only the processes of backing and epenthesis.

The study by Bowman, Parsons, and Morris (1984), which also reported phonological process use by children with DAS, has been reviewed previously in this chapter in sections dealing with error inconsistency and hypernasality.

In an attempt to determine the usefulness of the phonological approach to understanding the speech disorder of the children presenting DAS with whom we worked, Jackson and Hall (1987) addressed longitudinal change in use of phonological rules, using the *Compton-Hutton Phonological Assessment* (Compton & Hutton, 1978). Changes over time were found to occur in the two subjects' use of common and unique rules. Common rule use predominated and increased with age in the word initial position, while unique rule use decreased. It was noted that more rules, both common and unique, were written for errors in the sound classes of fricatives, affricates, liquids, and vocalics. However, the authors found individual variability in these trends.

In an additional study, Betsworth and Hall (1989) studied the application of phonological processes as defined by Stoel-Gammon and Dunn (1985) and Hodson and Paden (1983) by five subjects with DAS. They found that the process usage was highly individual. The subjects employed a total of 29 different processes and all five of the subjects used cluster reduction and gliding, as well as idiosyncratic processes which did not fall into the described categories. This study used two trials of the same stimulus words gathered on two different days. As discussed previously, the errors made on the same stimulus word were highly inconsistent leading to variability in the processes that described the error.

Variability was found in the results of the Jackson and Hall (1987) and Betsworth and Hall (1989) studies when phonological rules were applied to longitudinal data sets, as well as when applied to data gathered on two days close in time. This leads us to question the helpfulness of phonological analyses and the application of the theories underlying a phonological process approach to DAS because different views of a child's phonology could be gained if the testing was conducted on different days. For us, the motor control hypothesis better explains the inconsistencies and variabilities found in the speech of children with DAS.

Assessment

The clinician is cautioned that variability appears to be a factor that must be considered whether a phonological approach or a sound-by-sound approach is taken to analyze the speech of children with DAS. Some children with DAS may exhibit unique, idiosyncratic patterns. Other children may seem to exhibit patterns, although when the individual words on which the phonological analysis is based are examined, variability is revealed.

Prognosis

Perhaps one of the most frustrating aspects of DAS to professionals, as well as to the children and their families, is the very slow progress that is made despite what seems to be great amounts of remedial service and with good effort being expended on the part of the children themselves. As noted previously, slowness in improvement is cited by a number of authors in the literature (see Table 2.1).

The resistance of DAS to traditional or conventional remediation techniques has also been mentioned in the literature (see Table 2.1 for specific references). Unfortunately, research efforts systematically studying treatment effects for various types of remedial techniques with DAS are in their infancy. Discussions of selected remediation methods, as applied to children with DAS, will be discussed in Chapters 7, 8, and 9.

As speech-language professionals, we need to make major commitments of time to children with DAS. To cite Yoss and Darley (1974b), "these children require inordinate amounts of therapy time" (p. 24) and Rosenbek, Hansen, Baughman, and Lemme (1974) who stated that remedial "improvement was slow and inconsistent but persistent" (p. 20). Blakeley (1983) projected that 3 to 10 years of speech habilitation may be needed, and Aram (1980), stated that DAS patients she had followed had received 9 years of therapy. Air, Wood, and Neils (1989) stated that the remedial process was a long one for children with DAS "because usually each phoneme and consonant blend must be taught individually" (p. 274). The child described by Hall, Hardy, and LaVelle (1990) had received 12 years of services at the time of the report. Aram (1980) noted that while effectiveness of remediation could justifiably be questioned in some cases, "they are not children who move quickly in therapy, even in the best of hands" (p. 11).

What is the outcome for children with DAS? What will their speech be like when they are in high school? What will their speech sound like when they become adults?

Orton (1937) was the first to address prognosis in children he thought exhibited *developmental motor aphasia* or *motor speech delay*. He noted that the milder problems apparently resolved spontaneously but stated that a "certain measure of speech defect often persists in the form of a lisp or a defective /r/ or other infantilisms" (p. 120). Morley, Court, and Miller (1954) and later, Morley (1957, 1965, 1972) described prognosis from childhood through adulthood. She stated that spontaneous improvement was seen in many children and advocated therapy for children between the ages of 4 and 5, if intelligible speech had not been established by 4 years, so that the child could be understood when entering school. Morley further noted that in children with severe disabilities, the articulation disorder persisted into the adult years, describing a range of adult disorders from "minimal signs" to unintelligible. Ferry, Hall, and Hicks (1975) were more pessimistic in their prognostications, stating that "if intelligible speech has not developed by the age of 6 years, it is unlikely to develop" (p. 754). Aram (1980) described a group of children with DAS (number and severity unspecified) who ranged in ages from 3 to 14 years. She stated that none had achieved normal or even acceptable speech, although improvement had been seen in several members. Her impression was that the majority of the children with DAS would retain some articulatory and language deficits into adulthood. This prediction was based on the childrens' slow response in remediation and the continuing presence of communication disorders in adult members of their families. Making a similar observation was Blakeley (1983), who noted that as adults, children exhibiting DAS may continue to have difficulty in the production of words that are motorically complex. Weiss, Gordon, and Lillywhite (1987) stated that normal speech should not be expected except in the case of very mild "verbal dyspraxia." Further, "if the disorder is severe, then expect speech to be markedly impaired or even nonfunctional" (p. 266).

We have now followed several children with DAS into their high school and immediate post high school years, with one of these clients being described in the Hall, Hardy, and LaVelle (1990) study. Most of these clients continue to have some degree of difficulty, although this may reflect the generally severe disorders we see in our clinical setting. The children we follow receive a great deal of remedial assistance through their education agencies, the intensive program available through our clinic, or privately. With this help, most become functional oral communicators as they approach their late teen years. A few may even exhibit problems so minimal that the typical listener would not define any aspect of the communication system to be in error. However, upon very close examination, subtle voicing problems may be evident as well as a reduction of prosodic features, most notably the lack of pitch changes in inflections. They sound more monotonous than does the average speaker.

Our experience has indicated that, at least with those children with severe DAS, a "normal" outcome is unrealistic. As adults, these individuals may well be functional oral communicators but not "normal" ones. We also have certainly seen children exhibiting DAS who ultimately need to learn to use augmentative communication systems because of the severity of their problem and their response to intervention. For speech-language professionals, prognosis is an important issue with which to deal in the population of children with DAS. It is reflected in many quality-of-life issues such as vocational choices. Early counseling about possible outcome for children with severe DAS may help guide the child and their family in making informed and realistic vocational decisions.

Assessment

It is difficult to determine the prognosis for development of the articulation skills of a DAS child. Research in this area is nonexistent. Of necessity, the process is based on our own personal experience and those experiences shared by other professionals. As we approach this task, we often rely on multiple contacts with the child, watching and observing how the disordered speech sound system modifies with maturation and as a result of professional services.

There are multiple factors that influence our thinking about the eventual outcome of a DAS child's speech. One important factor is the severity of the DAS. However, this factor should not be the sole one on which a prognosis is made. Several other important factors will be addressed in more detail in following chapters. One is historical, the number of family members with communication disorders. Our experience has been that there may be a poorer prognosis when there are a number of close family members who have had or are experiencing similar types of problems. Another factor we use is the number and the severity of co-occurring problem areas such as language disorders, academic problems, and presence of oral apraxia. The child's cognitive functioning is another important aspect to consider as is the total educational program developed for the child.

One of the most telling factors, however, is the child's response to remediation to modify the articulation disorder that exists because of the apraxia. As will be discussed in Chapters 7, 8, and 9, this is an area in which little research has been conducted, so efficacy issues as to the most productive technique(s) or approach(es) are unknown at this time. Nonetheless, it has been our experience that the outcome is better for those children who begin receiving remedial services at an early age which directly addresses their speech sound problems. Likewise, the outcome seems more optimistic for those children who receive intervention on an intensive basis. However, the child's motivation, desire to communicate, and endurance to work with the speech-language professionals must also be considered.

The ramifications of the prognosis are great for the child with DAS. Thus, a prognosis should be carefully and thoughtfully considered and then carefully and thoughtfully shared with the family, and eventually, with the child.

CHAPTER 3

Theories of Motor Control: Descriptions, Issues, and Potential for Explaining DAS

We believe developmental apraxia of speech (DAS) is fundamentally a disorder of motor control. In an attempt to better understand the disorder, this chapter will describe selected theories of motor control and their potential for explaining DAS. Unfortunately, the relative dearth of information pertaining to theories of speech motor development and control inhibits our understanding of the effects of apraxia of speech in the developing organism. By contrast, there have been numerous attempts to explain acquired apraxia of speech in adults, where the most popularly held theories are derived from the literature on motor control. Because there is little information on developmental motor control for speech, we are forced to extrapolate from adult models to models that might be appropriate for children.

In this chapter, we will review briefly theories of motor control as they relate to apraxia of speech. We will also attempt to make inferences about the developing system, and by extension, offer possible explanations for DAS. The chapter will be devoted to an attempt to relate DAS to (1) possible neurologic bases, (2) selected theories of motor control, (3) issues related to the development of timing control, and (4) issues related to flexibility and plasticity in motor systems.

We offer this caveat: While we attempt to provide a theoretical basis for DAS, we are aware of no one theory that best accounts for the speech behaviors found in these children. Furthermore, none of the models or theories to be discussed have been tested rigorously enough with any subject group—normal or disordered, child or adult—to accept or reject them. Our purpose is to expose clinicians to a variety of theoretical approaches and share our current thoughts about the contribution of these models to a potential understanding of DAS. We hope this stimulates thinking in these areas to encourage data collection that tests the validity of any of these, or other, theories.

The remainder of this chapter will examine theories of motor control. We believe that it may help us to better understand DAS, if we examine those theories and speculate as to their potential for explaining the speech behaviors seen in DAS.

Theories of Motor Control and Their Relation to Apraxia of Speech

The first series of models to be described all assume that there is some form of motor programming that occurs during complex activities such as speech production. These models of programming have frequently been cited as relevant to explanations of acquired apraxia of speech in adults. The appeal of such an explanation for apraxia of speech in adults is readily apparent when one recalls Darley's (1968) original definition of the disorder as a disorder of "programming and sequencing" of speech units. As noted by Rosenbek, Kent, and LaPointe (1984) and Folkins (1985), the main problem with interpreting these models is the lack of agreement about the structure of a motor program. For instance, relevant features that are not typically identified in motor program models are the aspects of movement control that are programmed (e.g., velocity, amplitude, displacement). Moreover, the relevant features of a given motor program that are needed to perform a complex motor task are unknown. Nonetheless, selected theories of motor control may be instructive to us as speech clinicians and we will now review those theories. From time to time we will hypothesize about how these theories can be applied to work with clients with DAS.

Closed Loop Models

Models of speech production have used two different conceptual frameworks: a closed loop and an open loop. Review of these models can be found in Kent (1976) and their applicability to acquired apraxia of speech appears in Mlcoch and Noll (1980).

In brief, a closed loop model has three components: The first component comprises "effector units" (speech musculature), the second is a "feedback loop" which carries sensory information to the effector units, and the third is a "comparator" which compares speech output signals with an intended target. This model asserts that the control of speech relies on sensory feedback and assumes sensory information that exists as a result of speech production is fed back to the comparator. The comparator then makes a decision about whether the idealized target signal is the same as, or is different from, the output signal. If there is a discrepancy between the target and the actual output signal, an error signal is generated and used to correct the speech output. The error signal is the result of feedback. This process of comparison and correction may occur numerous times until a match between the target and output signal occurs. The production of errors explained by this model may originate within the feedback mechanism which is necessary to generate the original error signal. If the feedback mechanism is faulty, then the error signal may not serve its corrective functions and the motor system will not move correctly. Moreover, in this form, perhaps because of its brevity, the model fails to explain speech as other than a moment-to-moment series of independent actions and does not explain speech as a dynamic integrated process.

Modification of this model to include an associative chain expands the use of sensory information to facilitate speech production and attempts to recognize the dynamic nature of the speech production process. An associative chain assumes that any one movement within a series of movements, such as in speech, depends on information about whether a preceding movement has been completed. In the associative chain versus the closed loop model, perceptual information is utilized by the speech system to determine if movements associated with specific speech segments have been (1) initiated, (2) completed, and (3) produced correctly. If these three steps have been completed, the next segment is allowed to proceed. In order, then, for a second speech segment to proceed, the target and output signals must match. In this way, the model incorporates a sense of the dynamic nature of speech production in that the production of later speech segments depends on the accurate production of earlier occurring units.

One criticism of the closed loop associative chain model is that the time required for transmission of the sensory information produced by the speech production system to the central nervous system and then back to the peripheral musculature may be greater than 200 ms (Kent, 1976). Many segments of speech (e.g., consonants, formant transitions) occur more rapidly than this, and thus one would need to assume that the basic unit of speech is longer than the syllable. Mlcoch and Noll (1980) identified a second problem with this model: They noted that it does not account for contextual differences in speech production.

POTENTIAL FOR CLOSED LOOP MODEL TO EXPLAIN DAS. Errors in DAS might result from a number of different faulty mechanisms in the closed loop model. For instance, a problem with either the comparator or with the quality of the sensory information that is fed back to the system would result in an inadequately developed motor control system. As such, the movements for speech would be produced with difficulty and might be erroneous. This could result in the groping behavior often seen in children with DAS.

Another faulty mechanism in the model may be the failure of the motor programs to develop accurately. This might result in erroneous movements used for speech sound production. Deficits at this level of the model might result in substitutions of sounds as often seen in the speech of children with DAS. It is interesting to point out that a defect in the effector unit would result in a dysarthric error, not an apraxic error.

Examination of the associative chain model also offers some explanatory potential for certain errors found in DAS. Specifically, problems with the execution of the associative chain could result in sequencing problems. In the associative chain model, a speech segment cannot proceed until the previous movement has been completed, so speech segments that are allowed to proceed too soon will result in an inaccurate sequence of sounds. Additionally, if there are problems with the information in the chain about whether a segment has been completed or not, the initiation of speech may be hampered.

Open Loop Models

In contrast, open loop models generally postulate that sensory feedback is not necessary to execute normal speech. Rather, they posit that the speech movements are preprogrammed. Thus, these models imply a nervous system program, not unlike a computer program, in which the specific movements for speech segments are stored and carried out in a prewired fashion. Open loop systems do not have a mechanism for evaluation of the speech signal but comprise only the effector units (i.e., the speech musculature). The effector units respond to commands from some central input. Therefore, the effector units in open loop models do not rely on sensory information to perform accurate movements, but rather play out a predetermined neural code.

The critical features of the open loop model are: (1) the effector units, (2) the input signal (neural programs that drive the musculature), and (3) their interaction. The model assumes that the motor system has the ability to preset the effector unit before it receives an input signal. That is, the model assumes that there is knowledge about the musculature and that there are negligible disturbances of the movement pattern by outside influences (e.g., environmental constraints such as speaking situations, or sentence or phonemic context). There is no central comparator and no feedback mechanism. Thus, the input signal that arrives to the effector unit could be the same as the intended target or different from it because of a central problem or because of a transmission error. Because the effector unit is preset to receive only one type of input signal to trigger the program, it cannot correct an erroneous input signal.

The preprogramming model of Kent (1976), a version of the basic open-loop system, was developed to better understand the production of speech as a dynamic event. While the basic open loop model suggests that the intended motor commands are preset at the effector (muscle) level, the preprogramming model assumes that the commands that activate the muscle are not determined peripherally, rather they are specified by the central nervous system.

One criticism of open loop models is that it is unclear to us whether complex motor behaviors can occur without feedback. Moreover, it is difficult to imagine how an open loop system would function during development. It may be that, over time, the neuromotor system changes from primarily closed loop to primarily open loop. That is, at critical periods of motor development a closed loop system may be needed, but once specific movements for speech segments are stored, the system changes to an open-loop mechanism.

POTENTIAL FOR OPEN LOOP MODELS TO EXPLAIN DAS. Errors in speech sound production could be explained by open loop models in terms of faulty programming. Errors would not be related to faulty monitoring or correction since they are not provided by the model. For instance, if there were a faulty input signal, the effector unit would have to move according to that command and the output signal would be inaccurate. It does not seem as if this type of model has the potential to explain many of the symptoms seen in DAS, such as groping behavior, because the open loop model implies that the effector unit functions correctly or incorrectly without monitoring.

Serial Order Models

Rosenbek, Kent, and LaPointe (1984) also described serial order versions of motor program models. Serial order models are essentially open loop systems because they do not have a feedback mechanism. However, unlike the basic open loop model discussed above, serial order models attempt to explain the sequencing of movements as they occur in time.

In one version, based on Lashley's (1951) model of serial order in behavior, an attempt is made to relate movement to three stages of production: (1) determining tendency, (2) priming of expressive units, and (3) schema of order (see Kent, 1976). The determining tendency represents the idea to be expressed. The priming mechanism is used to alert the expressive language system and then select the appropriate linguistic units to be used in a given production. The schema of order places the selected units in the correct locations in an output unit. As noted by Rosenbek, Kent, and LaPointe (1984), the sequencing errors found in apraxic speakers might be accounted for by this model if the programs cannot be executed following the rules that define correct order in the speech system.

In motor programming's open loop form, authors (e.g., Semjen, 1977) have suggested that motor programs can be used to control the execution of lengthy sequences without feedback. As noted above, in the developing system it is highly unlikely that operations can occur without feedback from the various sensory systems. For any open loop programming model to work, one would have to assume an innate preprogramming of neurons. It seems unlikely that there is innate and complete preprogramming, given the need to learn individual speech sounds across different languages. Moreover, the amount of information that would need to be stored in a given motor program that functions without feedback would be so large that this form of the theory becomes implausible. A more moderate view of serial programming has suggested that programs can be executed but are subject to ongoing monitoring during speech production (e.g., Sternberg, Monsell, Knoll, & Wright, 1978). Such models may represent combined open and closed loop systems.

Roy's Hierarchical Model

Another form of the programming model was developed by Roy (1978) and is interesting to consider because it was specifically developed to account for apraxic errors seen in limb movements of adult patients with neurologic disease. However, because the data are based on experiments with the limbs, extrapolation of the model to the speech system must be necessarily guarded. Roy postulated that motor skill performance is based on hierarchically organized motor programs. The model has two major components: a "planner" and an "executor."

The planner comprises the goal selector and the sequencer. The highest level of Roy's model is the goal selector, which functions to select the goal for a given action. The model postulates that the goal selector is not operative for movements that are highly habituated. Thus, the more automatic a movement, the less it relies on the goal selector.

The next level of the system in Roy's model is the sequencer, which functions to order motor output. It has cognitive and perceptual components. The cognitive component makes decisions about effector units (musculature) and the sequencing of the movements. The perceptual component provides sensory information to assist in decision making by way of feedback loops.

The executor comprises a programmer, movement subroutines, and individual movement units. The programmer functions to work out the specifications derived from the planning component and programs the combinations of movements that will be required to accurately achieve a movement. The movement subroutines are programs that contain the various movements that need to be evoked to achieve a goal, while the individual movement units are single movements that make up a given pattern used by the subroutine component.

POTENTIAL FOR ROY'S HIERARCHICAL MODEL TO EXPLAIN DAS. Rosenbek, Kent, and LaPointe (1984) point out that an appeal of the hierarchical model is that it can account for errors at different levels of the speech production system. Faulty functioning of the planning component might give rise to the errors often found in the speech of children with DAS depending which component is involved. For instance, if the goal selector is not functioning properly, substitutions or distortions may occur because the exact movements needed for accurate speech might not be properly selected. On the other hand, errors in the sequencer might result in it being difficult to order speech sounds correctly. This difficulty in sequencing sounds could result in metathetic errors often described as being present in the speech of children with DAS. Moreover, it is possible that both components could be impaired, resulting in the variety of errors seen in DAS.

A poorly developed executer component might also give rise to speech errors observed in DAS. Defects in the programmer might be responsible for sound errors including omissions, substitutions, additions, and distortions. Problems with specific movement subroutines might give rise to distortions because the individual movement may not be selected properly. As well, sequencing errors might result from an error in the subroutines. Groping behaviors, when observed in children with DAS, could be the result of abnormal functioning of the perceptual component of the sequencer due to poor or faulty monitoring of ongoing speech.

Schema Theory

It is probable that some combined model, including both open and closed loop features, may most satisfactorily account for speech motor control and the errors made by apraxic speakers. One such model to be discussed is the schema theory (Schmidt, 1988) which was originally developed to explain motor control with no explicit attempt to extend the theory to speech production. As presented in 1975, Schmidt's theory postulates that there are three components of motor control systems: generalized motor program, recall schema, and recognition schema.

GENERALIZED MOTOR PROGRAM COMPONENT OF SCHEMA THEORY. According to Schmidt, a motor program is an abstract memory that, when activated, causes movement to occur. This program is similar to the one previously described for preprogrammed open loop systems. It suggests that the components of a movement are stored centrally and played out in much the same way a computer program operates. Thus, like an open loop system, there is a program that does not rely on feedback mechanisms to operate or to execute a movement. However, unlike purely open loop models, in schema theory, there are numerous ways to execute a generalized motor program.

In the generalized motor program, various movement parameters (e.g., force, velocity, displacement) are determined prior to execution. The program contains some abstract notion of which components make up a movement, but the actual physiological variables that are employed for a given task may vary. It is thought that this provides a way to use one generalized motor program for a variety of different tasks.

RECALL SCHEMA COMPONENT OF SCHEMA THEORY. The second part of Schmidt's schema theory involves the use of recall schema in response production. A recall schema is defined as a rule based on past experience (i.e., related to previous attempts to achieve the movement goal). The development of recall schema requires information pertaining to the initial conditions used to execute a given movement such as specific physiological parameters, relative positions of structures, and knowledge of the results. A logical extension of this premise is that the greater the number of experiences with a given generalized motor program, the more developed are the recall schema.

RECOGNITION SCHEMA COMPONENT OF SCHEMA THEORY. The third component of Schmidt's schema theory addresses recognition schema, which are used for evaluation of the target response. Recognition schema comprise initial conditions, past and current outcomes of movements, and the sensory consequences of actions. As additional variability is encountered with a given task, the scope of the recognition schema is expanded. This expansion increases the strength of the recognition schema, which is also enhanced by expanding knowledge of results. Evaluation of a movement may occur during the production of movements and/or after its completion. Outcomes of novel responses may be predicted because their development is dependant on the variability of past experiences.

SCHEMA THEORY AND DEVELOPMENT OF MOTOR SKILLS. One tenet of Schmidt's schema theory is the need for experience of variability during the production of movements. Thus, the more opportunities to perform a movement under different conditions, the stronger the recall and recognition schema. Shapiro and Schmidt (1982) reported that schema development occurs more easily in children than in adults. They noted that normal children show greater achievement in performing a movement task when they have experienced variable practice and learn the skill better than adults who have similar amounts and types of practice.

A factor to be considered in the development of motor skills relates to criterion practice versus varied practice of a skill. During criterion practice, subjects are asked to practice on the specific skill that is being developed. By contrast, during varied practice, subjects receive the same amount of practice but practice on novel tasks. The variable practice condition typically elicits greater performance skill than does practice on the specific task itself. Shapiro and Schmidt (1982) suggest that skill transfer to a novel task is related to the amount of variable practice a subject receives. Thus, skill transfer is increased with greater amounts of variable practice.

SCHEMA THEORY AND KNOWLEDGE OF RESULTS (KR). According to Schema theory, "knowledge of results (KR)" is important in the development of motor control. KR may be useful in understanding how motor skills might be independently acquired, as well as being instructive in terms of teaching motor skills with all populations. KR is extrinsic feedback (information about achievement of a task in regard to the environmental goal) and consists of information about the outcome of a movement. Schmidt (1988) stresses that it is not information about the movement itself that has been termed "knowledge of performance (KP)" which will be discussed later in the chapter.

The temporal relation between the time when a movement is performed and the time when KR is provided may affect motor learning. Figure 3.1 illustrates the paradigm used to experimentally study the temporal relationship of KR and movements. After a movement has been performed (R_1 in the figure), there is a delay until KR is given. This delay is called the *KR-delay interval.* Then KR is given (KR_1 in the figure speci-

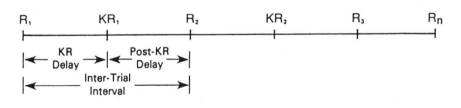

FIGURE 3.1. Temporal placement of events in the KR paradigm. *Note.* From *Motor Control and Learning,* 2nd ed., by R. A. Schmidt, 1988, Champaign, IL: Human Kinetics. Copyright 1988 by Richard A. Schmidt. Reprinted by permission.

fies that the KR is for the first response). There is then a period of time before the next movement is performed (R_2 in the figure). This time period between KR and a subsequent response is termed the *post-KR delay*. Results of studies examining the KR-delay interval have shown that the length of this interval makes little difference in the acquisition of skilled movements (Schmidt 1988; Salmoni, Schmidt, & Walter, 1984).

The use of "filled" versus "empty" KR-delay intervals impacts on the amount of learning of motor skills that can occur. If the KR-delay interval is filled with movements not related to the task at hand, there is a negative effect on performance of a targeted task (Shea & Upton, 1976). While Marteniuk (1986) has argued that this decrease in performance, associated with a filled interval, is related to a "high-level planning process," Schmidt (1988) has argued that it is constrained by the limits of short-term memory. An alternative explanation may be that the interfering task draws from the attentional resources allocated to the task and diminishes the available attentional capacity with the result that the person cannot attend sufficiently to the incoming KR for it to be maximally beneficial.

Regardless of the reason, we believe the practical implications are clear: Keep the KR-delay interval empty. During therapy activities for children with DAS, this suggests that one should not talk to the child during this interval. Moreover, the clinical session should be structured such that during this interval no other activities are occurring. Note that this interval is thought of as occurring in a short time period after the KR and before the next attempt. If this interval is too long, it may be detrimental to task performance and learning.

During the next interval, the post-KR-delay interval, the subject is an active processor of information. The subject has time to think about the movement and the preceding KR that has been provided. That is, KR has been delivered and this information must be assimilated and remembered for use. In the case of an error, the subject must respond to the KR to change the movement pattern on succeeding trials (R_2 in Figure 3.1). If the interval between KR and a response allows for active processing of information, then one expects that the length of the post-KR-delay interval is critical in achieving maximal performance. If this delay is too short, there is not enough time for the person to put the information into memory. This will have a negative affect on the next attempt to respond and thereby on subsequent learning of the specific skill. On the other hand, filling the post-KR-delay interval severely degrades performance on motor tasks (Schmidt, 1988), suggesting that this interval is crucial in overall learning.

The aforementioned information about the post-KR-delay interval may have important ramifications for the structuring of therapy sessions with children who have DAS. Clinicians should be aware of the effects of filling the post- KR-delay interval with instructions or other verbal information to the child. Time is needed for the child to process the response and the subsequent KR in order for learning to occur. However, filling the post-KR-delay interval may be used advantageously to assess the stability of the speech sound skills. If the interval is filled, and a performance decrement results, then one can assume that the skill is not stable and needs continued remedial efforts.

A different situation emerges when KR is given after a number of responses as opposed to the one response as illustrated above. Figure 3.2 illustrates the paradigm in which the KR for a response is given after many responses have occurred. As shown in the figure, the KR for each of the many responses is delayed. This method, described by Bilodeau (1956, 1966, 1969), has been termed *trials-delay*. A subject might receive KR_1 after R_3 and KR_2 after R_5 and so on. As trial delay increases, performance decreases. This type of delayed extrinsic feedback has been shown to be extremely detrimental to motor learning and should be avoided. In our opinion, during treatment of speech problems of children with DAS, reinforcement schedules should take note of this type of KR and be careful to avoid its use.

Some researchers have compared immediate KR (after every trial) to summary KR (feedback given after a selected number of responses). Schmidt (1988) writes that immediate KR may be detrimental to performance while summary KR may be helpful. His interpretation is that immediate KR provides a subject with too much information. It is also the case that immediate KR disrupts the post-KR-delay interval, which also hampers learning. One must be careful to consider the optimum number of trials to be summarized. An example of a nonspeech task used to study this was to have a subject move a ball up a tube by blowing air through a pipe below the ball. Schmidt (1988) has noted that the most effective number of trials to summarize in giving KR, in this paradigm, is 5. Fewer trials ($n = 1$) or more trials ($n = 10$) degraded performance and were not as effective in learning a new skill.

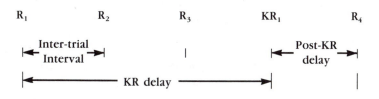

FIGURE 3.2. Placement of events during summary KR.

SCHEMA THEORY AND KNOWLEDGE OF PERFORMANCE (KP). Information about the movement, not the environmental goal, is termed knowledge of performance. This type of information is directed toward the movement pattern. Schmidt (1988) notes that this type of feedback may be related to aspects of a complex movement that a person is only vaguely aware of even aspects of movements that they cannot be consciously aware of such as that provided by biofeedback. This type of feedback ranges from somewhat vague comments about a movement to quite complex reports in which the subject is provided with detailed information about various aspects of the movement (e.g., during limb movement tasks one might say "you missed the target by 2 inches," while during speech remediation one might say "your tongue was too far to the left for correct production of that sound").

While KP is effective in teaching motor skills, one must be careful in how much information is presented. Too much diverse information, particularly when training a complex motor skill, may result in a situation in which the learner does not know what information is most important (Schmidt, 1988). Thus, the learner will become bogged down in the details and not develop and/or refine the skill. In terms of teaching speech production skills to children with DAS, this seems a noteworthy caution. It suggests that we must be very careful in the amount and type of feedback we give the children, and that we might need to approach the remediation of a speech sound in terms of successive approximations. By making the initial goal less than perfection, we can limit the amount of information provided and maintain a high level of success. As goals are achieved, the criteria for acceptance are narrowed, thereby maintaining an appropriate amount of feedback information while progressing toward more accurate sound production.

Prior to discussing the implications of schema theory to help understand DAS, a note of caution is needed. Most of the data on schema theory have been gathered in experimental contexts, which, by necessity, makes them artificial and only indirectly applicable to real life situations. Moreover, the studies were not aimed at understanding speech motor skill acquisition and generalization to speech may not be entirely appropriate. Nevertheless, we believe that the insights about motor learning provided by such studies are instructive to us as speech clinicians, and this information may be useful in structuring therapy sessions.

POTENTIAL FOR SCHEMA THEORY TO EXPLAIN DAS. As an explanation of DAS, schema theory might suggest that the speech errors made by children with DAS may be the result of breakdown at any one of, or any combination of, the previously specified levels of motor execution and control (i.e., generalized motor programs, recall schema, and recognition schema). An inability to develop accurate or complete generalized motor programs might result in difficulty executing speech movements accurately. The movements that result in a given sound production would be faulty.

Given an accurate generalized motor program, poorly developed recall or recognition schema might also result in the speech errors observed in DAS. For example, if the rules (recall schema) that activate a motor program are faulty or poorly developed, then the production of articulator movements would be similarly faulty or incomplete. This could result in sound substitutions, additions, or distortions, depending on the stability of the rule. Furthermore, generalized motor programs might be erroneous as continued development and adjustments occur. This implies that the information feeding back to the motor program is inaccurate.

On the other hand, a deficit in the recognition schema might interfere with the ongoing monitoring of movement accuracy. The groping behaviors seen in children with DAS might well be the result of insufficient monitoring of movement accuracy. Errors in the recognition schema might also give rise to poor predictability of movement outcome in novel situations. This could result in a situation where different phonetic contexts would create more errors in the speech of the child exhibiting DAS.

One might hypothesize that the groping behaviors observed in DAS are related to poorly developed recognition schema, while the actual production errors themselves may be associated with abnormal or slow development of recall schema. Unique speech errors, such as those described in children with DAS (see Chapter 2), might result from an inability to correctly predict outcome in different environments due to poorly developed recognition schema.

A further complication for the child with developmental apraxia accounted for by the schema theory is that the normal development of the motor system depends on practice and experience. Given that the child with DAS has fewer successful experiences with speech, and repetition, practice, and reinforcement are necessary to acquire and develop motor programs—recall schema and recognition schema may be impoverished. For example, the child with few successes with speech may become increasingly nonverbal due to a lack of experiences that limit reinforcement and result in a failure to develop motor programs. This may also be a useful concept to help explain "lost" sounds which will be described Chapter 4. Therefore, the components of the motor response are less well developed, because of lack of practice, in the child with DAS than in the normal speaking child. It follows that extensive practice and drill work would be reasonable therapeutic approaches if this theoretical approach is valid.

In developing practice routines and using "drill" activities during remediation, one must decide when to give KR and how much information to provide the child. As well, care must be taken to fill, or not to fill, the various intervals.

Development and Control of Timing

While the models discussed thus far are theoretically based, they clearly provide a potential explanatory framework for the genesis of the speech errors found in children with DAS. Nevertheless, there remain other areas to be discussed that also impact on speech production and, by extension, to DAS. One such aspect of motor development is the control of timing. Temporal (timing) factors are critical in the development of motoric systems. The precise control of timing is crucial for the accurate production of speech in that there are aspects of the speech production that require a highly precise timing mechanism (e.g., the onset of voicing and the length of specific sound segments). The hypothesis that apraxia of speech (in adults) may be a disorder of temporal coordination (cf., Itoh, Sasanuma, & Ushijuma, 1979; Kelso & Tuller, 1981) appears to be particularly relevant to the discussion of timing control in motor systems and timing problems in children with DAS. However, there is little empirical evidence that addresses this issue. It appears that to achieve accurate motor skill performance, timing must be controlled relative to information obtained from the environment. In speech, the movement goals may need to be coordinated with outside events (e.g., the social or linguistic context in which one produces speech) as well as with the surrounding phonemes in the target production.

The development of timing also may be related to mechanisms intrinsic to the individual. That is, the timing of various aspects of speech production (respiration, phonation, resonance, and articulation) must be coordinated with one another within the system and between the systems. Timing for accurate speech production appears to depend on both motoric and perceptual contributions.

Components of both open and closed loop models have included aspects of timing behavior in the performance of motor skills. As noted by Wade (1982), these models imply that sensory and motor nerves are independent and are separated by an error-correcting device that regulates the timing between these two systems. In regard to development, Wade (1982) suggests that timing accuracy, at least for nonspeech motor skills, improves over time. Wade's study, in which children were to strike a target moving from the left to the right, indicates that normal children between the ages of 7 to 14 years show decreased variability when performing these tasks that require fairly precise timing skills.

Wade postulated that a critical factor in the development of temporal components of movement is the "response formulation." He hypothesized that individuals' interactions with the environment drive the development of the temporal components of the motor system. Such development depends on perceptual information received from the environment.

The performance of motor skills related to limb movements requires visual and tactile/kinesthetic information. The development of timing, in regard to speech production, probably requires perceptual information derived from the auditory and tactile/kinesthetic systems. With respect to perceptual information, it is known that the auditory system is an extremely finely tuned temporal integrator (Robin & Royer, 1987). Adults are able to detect a gap of less than 2 ms between two tones (Yost & Nielsen, 1977). Data on normal children suggest that temporal acuity improves between the ages of 7 and 14 years (McCroskey, 1984).

In summary, it is evident that timing control in both motoric and perceptual systems appears to improve throughout childhood. It is also clear that perceptual information about timing is needed to refine timing control during the performance of motor tasks. To our knowledge, these studies have not been extended into adulthood.

Potential for Errors of Timing to Explain DAS

If children exhibiting developmental apraxia have difficulty with the control of movements because of aberrant timing, one might predict certain speech production problems such as voicing errors due to poor coordination of timing between the phonatory and articulatory systems. In addition, poor control of timing of the movements of the articulators could result in abnormal speech sound production, such as the distortion of vowels, inappropriate nasal production, or production of unusual non-phonemic errors observed in children with DAS. Other problems with timing might be reflected in a reduction of speech rate or abnormalities in prosodic features of speech. For instance, the lengthening of words serves in some instances to signal stress in a sentence context. The child with DAS, who has difficulty controlling timing, might produce inappropriate stress allocation within sentences.

Flexibility and Variability in Motor Control

The issues of flexibility and variability in motor control have been described in detail by Folkins (1985). In discussing these issues, Folkins described an integrated approach to motor control in which holistic behavioral goals (perceptually accurate speech) need to be targeted, as opposed to defining the speech goals in terms of individual segments such as phonetic units. This holistic approach is quite different from those discussed above yet it has both intuitive and scientific appeal. In Folkins' view, the intent of the speaker is to produce "perceptually adequate" speech output. As such, the motor system of an individual speaker must develop motor strategies for the motor system from a rules designed to achieve the perceptual goal. Folkins argues that in this model there is no need to assume that the speech motor system is constrained by phonetic units. This approach suggests that there may be numerous ways for the motor system to implement the rules, and these may vary between speakers and within a speaker from context to context.

Folkins notes that when a speaker is asked to repeat the same speech sample, there can be variations along many different physiological parameters (e.g., velocity, displacement) without changing the perceived speech output. The *flexible* variations that occur when a speech sample is repeated reflect the ability of the motor system to still reach the same goal with variation in the individual physiological parameters. Folkins writes that there are two types of flexibility. In the case noted above, where the same speech sample is repeated, the motor system is demonstrating *free-variation flexibility*. This refers to the ability of the individual physiological parameters of the motor system to be interchanged without cost. This concept might be related to the development of motor programs discussed earlier (see Schema Theory p. 56) which require variability to complete development. The ability to vary physiological parameters in various ways while producing the same speech sample may be a means by which motor programs are developed and strengthened over time. The amount of displacement or the speed of movement of speech structures may vary from sample to sample, but the perception of the speech produced remains the same.

Folkins termed the second type of flexibility *forced flexibility,* which refers to the situation where the speaking conditions change. In this case, the motor system is flexible enough to have its physiological parameters altered to achieve the desired speech output goal, even though the conditions under which the sample is uttered have changed. Experimentally this type of flexibility has been observed during the placement of a bite-block to fix the jaw during speech production. Another example of forced flexibility is when a phoneme is produced in different phonetic contexts. Here the various physiological parameters may vary because of the context, but the phoneme produced maintains its perceptual accuracy. Both of these concepts of flexibility are clearly important because speakers, including children with DAS, need to be able to modify various parameters of speech production during ongoing speech due to the changing demands of a given situation or specific message.

There are also situations, according to Folkins (1985), in which speakers are forced to modify the parameters of speech because of pathologies of the speech production system. These situations are not addressed by the flexibility discussed above. For example, structural alterations of the speech mechanism (e.g., oral trauma or orthodontia) require the speaker to adjust to this new condition. In such cases, the speaker may have the ability to modify the rule system that drives the musculature to achieve acceptable speech. Folkins refers to this ability to change the rule system as "plasticity." As with the establishment of the initial rule system, eventual modification of an existing system requires time. Furthermore, these rule changes are relatively permanent as compared to the temporary changes in physiological parameters related to flexibility. It is important to realize that there are obvious limitations to the amount of flexibility or plasticity an individual is capable of demonstrating, and when these limitations are exceeded, errors will result.

In summary, in order to understand the variability within the speech motor system, Folkins (1985) has proposed several types of "interactions" that can account for changes in the parameters of speech production which result in perceptually acceptable speech. *Type Ia interaction* refers to free-variation flexibility and represents changes in physiologic parameters that occur when the same speech sample is repeated in the same context. *Type Ib interaction* refers to forced-variation flexibility which represents changes in physiologic parameters as a result of physical factors. *Type II interaction* refers to plasticity, which is the speaker's ability to modify the rule system over time.

Potential of Flexibility and Variability to Explain DAS

The types of variability discussed above may be helpful in understanding children with DAS. Most descriptions of apraxia of speech, whether they refer to the acquired form or the developmental form, address the variability of performance as a distinguishing feature. In the literature dealing with acquired apraxia of speech in adults, there have been a number of physiologic studies that allow consideration of the issues of variability and flexibility to be examined. For example, Itoh, Sasanuma, and Ushijuma (1979) observed that the displacement of the timing between the lowering of the velum and the elevation of the tongue tip for the production of /d/ were poorly coordinated in an apraxic speaker compared to a normal speaker. It may be that the physiological variations of temporal incoordination of displacement represent Type II interactions. As a result, the apraxic speaker has modified his rule system following cerebral insult, and the changes do not represent a defect in a physiologic parameter, per se.

Application of this theoretical viewpoint to developmental apraxia of speech may be fruitful. One must first decide whether children with DAS might be viewed as having forced-variation flexibility (a Type Ib interaction). Problems with one or more parameters of speech motor control (e.g., velocity, timing, force control) might result in the speech symptoms in DAS. If this assumption is correct, the child with DAS can be thought of as having reduced forced-variation flexibility is some instances and will need to modify existing motor rules, or develop new ones, to compensate for these problems.

However, modification of motor rules because of a forced variation may come with a cost to the speaker. This cost may, or may not, be so great as to disrupt speech. We postulate that the cost to a child demonstrating DAS, when contrasted to a normal speaking child, might be large enough to disrupt accurate speech production. Thus, the cost to the child with DAS results in a situation in which that child may be less efficient at producing accurate speech than the normally developing child. Therefore, the child exhibiting DAS may have less flexibility to use when stress is placed on the motor speech system. This inefficiency could result in performance with highly variable error patterns, as well as a greater tendency to demonstrate breakdowns in speech production when communicative complexity increases.

As noted in Chapter 2, children exhibiting DAS have been reported to be inconsistent in their speech. This inconsistency has often been observed perceptually. We would suggest that inconsistency in the speech of children with DAS results from lack of the variability used by the motor system to produce speech movements. Such variability may result in inconsistent speech such that one may observe (1) moments of error-free speech, that then breaks down and (2) different errors during the production of the same sound.

Summary

We have reviewed some major motor theories and attempted to show the potential each of these theories has to explain the speech errors made by children with DAS. None of the theories have previously been suggested or yet been demonstrated to account for DAS. Critical elements of the disorder may also be addressed by issues of the control of timing and flexibility/variability of the speech motor system. Changes in the developing motor speech system may result in modifications of the motor rules used to implement speech acts. Such modification, for the child with DAS, may result in problems related to the accurate and consistent production of phonemes.

CHAPTER 4

Language and Academic Learning Problems: Co-occurring Characteristics of Children Exhibiting DAS

C hildren with developmental apraxia of speech seldom experience problems with only their speech production. Frequently they exhibit problems in other areas as well. While the focus of this book is on the articulatory speech behavior of children with DAS, we think it is imperative that professionals working with children exhibiting DAS be aware of, and respond to, other factors that contribute to making the individual child with DAS the child with whom we deal. While these factors may not necessarily be central to the *speech* problems of the child, we acknowledge that they frequently co-occur with the speech production difficulties experienced by a child with DAS. We believe strongly that we must address the total needs of the child with DAS and not focus only on the apraxic component of the disordered communication process. Some of these factors, or characteristics, affect how we directly manage the child with DAS, while others will influence how we work as a member of a team of professionals concerned about a child with DAS. In this chapter, we will discuss language and educational issues that often must be addressed when working with a child with DAS.

Many of the children demonstrating DAS whom we have seen in our clinic present aberrant language development and later, disordered skills in all language domains. In addition, they may exhibit academic learning difficulties. *At this time,* the interactions among the apraxic speech, the language disorders, and the academic learning difficulties are unclear. That is, the effects of speech production problems on language learning and academic learning have not been definitively studied. Thus we consider any disorders in the language domains to be concomitant, or to co-exist, with the DAS. Our discussions of these areas will be accompanied by tables that contain citations and synopses of relevant studies and reports from the literature. The tables also contain information for each study about the number of reported children we presume exhibited DAS versus how many of those children with DAS exhibited the specific characteristic

addressed in the table. We emphasize again that much of the DAS literature involves single case studies or small numbers of subjects/clients,
which needs to be considered when drawing overall conclusions about
the larger population of children with DAS.

Delayed Development of Oral Communication Skills

There are frequent reports of delayed oral expressive speech and/or
delayed language skills in the developmental histories of children with
DAS. Hadden's 1891 case description reflects this delay with the report
that Charles M. first started to produce speech sounds during his third
year of life, which is beyond the age range when speech is first expected
to occur. However, delays in the development of oral communication
may not be exhibited by all children with DAS. For instance, 7 of the
12 children reported by Morley (1957, 1959, 1965, 1972) were reported
to have had normal speech and/or language development. Nevertheless,
the literature (Table 4.1) suggests that delayed speech and language development occurs, particularly in children with severe DAS involvement.

The differences between the child who is later diagnosed as exhibiting
DAS and their normal peers may be evident in early infancy as is revealed
in reports of preverbal behavior. Johnson and Myklebust (1967) reported
that children with *verbal apraxia* were silent babies and did not babble
as much as other children in their families. Eisenson (1972) reported that
infants who were later diagnosed as exhibiting *congenital articulatory
apraxia* did not engage in vocal play, echolalia, or verbal imitation. Lohr
(1978) also addressed the lack of infant verbal play behaviors, reporting
that the five children she followed were quiet babies who did not babble.
She also noted that their early vocalizations did not develop into differentiated speech sounds. Other authors describe similar lack of infant vocal/
verbal development. Aram and Glasson (1979) reported not only quiet
babies but a lack of babbling as well. Harlan (1984) also noted a quiet
baby in his case report, while Hall, Hardy and LaVelle (1990) noted a lack
of cooing and babbling with their presented case.

Parental reports of the children with DAS we have followed frequently include reports of "quiet," or even "silent" babies, who do little,
if any, cooing or babbling. In fact, this characteristic seems to be so notable
and unique to the developmental histories of children exhibiting DAS that
when this is reported, it flags for us a possible DAS hypothesis during
the diagnostic process. We have also noted that these quiet or silent babies
are often reported to be "good" babies, causing us to question if there
may be an interaction between the lack of infant noise and parental perceptions in the ease of infant care. We also have noted that parents frequently say that they initially became concerned about their child's
speech-language development sometime between the child's first and

TABLE 4.1
Development of Oral Communication Skills in Children with DAS

REFERENCE	NUMBER OF PRESUMED CHILDREN WITH DAS REPORTED TO HAVE DELAYED SPEECH AND/OR LANGUAGE DEVELOPMENT	MANIFESTATIONS OF DELAYED OR DEVIANT SPEECH AND/OR LANGUAGE DEVELOPMENT
Hadden, 1891	1/1	"Did not speak at all until he was between 3 and 4 years old when he began to make sounds" (p. 96)
Orton, 1937	Not reported	"Most children in this group are late in beginning to talk" (p. 119)
Morley, 1957, 1959, 1965, 1972	5/12	Mean age for production of: First word—19 months Phrases—33 months
Walton, Ellis, & Court, 1962	3/3	Subject VP "used words from the age of 2½ years, gradually acquired sentences" (p. 604) Subject DL "By 15 months he was using words & phrases, but at 18 months he had a severe case of tonsillitis without apparent neurological complications, and did not begin to speak easily again until his 4th year" (p. 605) Subject DN used single words at 2 years, used sentences at 2½ years
Johnson & Myklebust, 1967	Not reported	Silent babies Do not babble as much as other children in family

(Continued)

TABLE 4.1   (Continued)

REFERENCE	NUMBER OF PRESUMED CHILDREN WITH DAS REPORTED TO HAVE DELAYED SPEECH AND/OR LANGUAGE DEVELOPMENT	MANIFESTATIONS OF DELAYED OR DEVIANT SPEECH AND/OR LANGUAGE DEVELOPMENT
Eisenson, 1972	Not reported	As infants the children engage in little vocal play, verbal imitation, or echolalic activities Continues to be nonverbal despite gains in comprehension
Rosenbek & Wertz, 1972	50/50	Delayed or abnormal speech development
Lohr, 1978	5/5	Quiet babies No babbling Vocalizations did not develop into differentiated speech sounds
	4/5	"Lost" words
Aram & Glasson, 1979	8/8	Mean age for onset: Single words—2.9 years 2-word phrases—4.2 years
	4/8	Quiet babies Did not babble as expected
Crary, 1984a	17/25	Age at speech onset was over 2 years of age
	2/25	Normal speech development until 2 years, then regressed
Harlan, 1984	1/1	Quiet baby
Love & Fitzgerald, 1984	1/1	Delayed language and phonologic skills
Riley, 1984	7/15	Abnormal language development Delayed onset of sentences
Hall, 1989	1/1	Prolonged use of single utterance Slow development of word combinations at 7 years of age

(Continued)

TABLE 4.1 (Continued)

REFERENCE	NUMBER OF PRESUMED CHILDREN WITH DAS REPORTED TO HAVE DELAYED SPEECH AND/OR LANGUAGE DEVELOPMENT	MANIFESTATIONS OF DELAYED OR DEVIANT SPEECH AND/OR LANGUAGE DEVELOPMENT
Hall, Hardy, & LaVelle, 1990	1/1	No cooing or babbling First word reported at 4 years of age 2-word combinations at 7 years of age

second birthdays, as the child failed to make appropriate growth in oral expressive skills. However, the parents may not have actively sought help at that time.

As the child with DAS grows and develops physically, a delayed pattern is frequently evident in relation to later developing milestones in speech and language development. A child's first word is viewed as a significant event in that child's life. Unfortunately, for the parents of a child with DAS, the wait for this event is often a long one. Studies have addressed this issue, although the criteria used to define *first word* is usually not specified. Hadden (1891) reported that Charles M. did not speak until he was between 3 and 4 years old. Morley (1957, 1959) cited 19 months as the mean age for the production of the first word with the five children she diagnosed as having *articulatory dyspraxia,* while Aram and Glasson (1979) cited 2.9 years as the mean age for their eight children with DAS. Case studies have reported varying, but delayed, ages for the occurrence of the first word and include 2.5 years for subject VP and 2 years for subject DN (Walton, Ellis & Court, 1962); over 2 years of age (Crary, 1984a); and 4 years of age (Hall, Hardy & LaVelle, 1990).

Likewise, the combination of words into phrases and sentences is also heralded as a significant milestone in speech and language development. Morley (1957, 1959, 1965, 1972) reported the mean age for this was 33 months in her group of five children with DAS, while Aram and Glasson (1979) reported the mean age for the utterance of two-word phrases was 4.2 years. Hall, Hardy, and LaVelle (1990) reported two-word combinations first occurred at 7 years of age with the child described in their case study.

The reports made by the parents of children with DAS we follow corroborate the literature citations of delayed acquisition of important speech and language skills. In addition, we have had the unique opportunity to follow a number of children with DAS over time, allowing us to examine the development of their communication skills. The Jackson and Hall (1987) study discussed in Chapter 3 examined, longitudinally, the development of speech sound skills in four children with DAS. The results suggest that the childrens' acquisition of sound classes, phonological rules, and types of articulatory errors followed normal developmental patterns, although this development was delayed. The children with DAS acquired articulatory proficiencies at slower rates and at older ages than did children with no problems in their articulatory development. However, it must be understood that the children involved in the study had received intensive remedial assistance and exhibited a number of the DAS characteristics (including inconsistencies) while these normal patterns of acquisition were occurring. While, over time, the gross acquisition patterns followed a normal course, each child's path was highly variable, probably due to the DAS. As was discussed in Chapter 2, it must be understood that *normal* articulation skills are not the probable outcome for these four children.

Assessment

We think that it is important to obtain a case history documenting, via the reports of parent(s) or guardian, the development of the child's communication system. We have found that many parents of children in whom we suspect DAS are able to recall specific ages when skills were acquired because the ages were much older than the parents thought was normal, or usual, or the skill had been so long awaited. The use of baby books, home videos, or other memorabilia also may help document development. It is also useful to explore all language domains, both as the language developed and current functional use. Remember to strive for estimates of the child's receptive skills as well as expressive ones. From this background information, the speech-language clinician can gain an appreciation of the developmental course the child has taken, as well as a sense of parental concerns and needs.

Unique Aspects of Communication Development

There are reports of several somewhat unique aspects in the struggle of children with DAS to develop expressive oral skills. One is the prolonged use of a single utterance to convey multiple word meanings. A client in our clinic was reported to use the reduplicated syllable /gaga/ in such a manner (Hall, 1989). A similar use of a single utterance was also reported by Lohr (1978).

A second unique aspect in communication skill development of children with DAS, and one that is particularly distressing to their parents, is the "loss" of words. This was reported by Walton, Ellis, and Court (1962) to have occurred with Subject DL, whom they had diagnosed as exhibiting articulatory apraxia. Although DL was reported to have been using words and phrases by the age of 15 months, the subject ceased talking at 18 months when he was reported to have had a severe case of tonsillitis "without apparent neurological complications" (p. 605). The child "did not begin to speak easily again until his 4th birthday" (p. 605). Crary (1984a) reported that 2 of the 25 children he diagnosed as exhibiting *developmental verbal dyspraxia* regressed in their speech development after the age of 2 years. Lohr (1978) also noted that words became "lost" to children with *verbal apraxia.*

In our clinical practice, we have not received reports of children exhibiting DAS regressing in overall verbal skill levels for protracted periods of time. However, like Lohr, we have had a number of parents report the loss of a word. Parents become very frustrated and anxious when, after their child seems able to produce a word, they lose it, being unable to even approximate the former production. To quote the parent of one of our clients: "The words just seem to evaporate and never return." This phenomenon also occurs in the remedial process in the form of a lost phoneme or word; fortunately, it has been our experience that the loss is usually regained. This aspect of communication acquisition may be part of the inconsistency and variability that characterize DAS. For example, a preschooler seen in our clinic, who was successful for some time with production of /p/ in syllables, suddenly was unable to produce it, substituting the voiced cognate /b/ instead. The /p/ sound was probed during a number of sessions, without success, until during one session, he was once again able to produce it correctly in syllables, continuing to make progress with the phoneme after that time. This may be an example of inconsistency in the form of a lost phoneme that is later regained.

A third example of unique characteristics, particularly of children with severe DAS involvement, is the use of gestures and other non-speech methods of communicating. Reports of this in the literature are summarized in Table 4.2. Inspection of the Table reveals that the children are inventive in the development of nonverbal communication systems. The upper limbs are most frequently cited as used in nonverbal communication, ranging from pointing, pulling, gesturing, using "crude gesture systems", and forms of sign language. The use of non-speech "mouth noises" is also cited in the literature, with descriptions of vocalizations, onomatopoeic sounds, and grunting.

TABLE 4.2

Reports of Use of Gestures and Nonverbal Vocalizations by Children with DAS

REFERENCE	NUMBER OF PRESUMED CHILDREN WITH DAS REPORTED TO USE GESTURES AND VOCALIZATIONS	COMMENTS
Hadden, 1891	1/1	Expressed "his wants by nodding or shaking his head or by pointing" (p. 96)
Orton, 1937	Not Reported	"They use their hands freely in pointing to objects to obtain their desires, but we have never seen any indication of the development of true symbolic gestures as in a sign language" (p. 119)
McGinnis, Kleffner, & Goldstein, 1956	Not Reported	"The child usually relies on gestures to convey meanings" (p. 240)
Johnson & Myklebust	Not Reported	Severely involved nonverbal children with "verbal apraxia" "communicate largely by gesture and pantomime" (p. 123)
Hunter, 1975	Not Reported	"In the extreme, these children relied on a crude gesture system for communication" (p. 130)
Lohr, 1978	NR/5	Used vocalization, gestures, and other nonvocal cues
Aram & Glasson, 1979	NR/8	Used gestures and onomatopoeic sounds
Harlan, 1984	1/1	"Expression characterized by . . . pointing, pulling, and gesturing" (p. 122)
Love & Fitzgerald, 1984	1/1	"Communication usually consisted of . . . hand gestures" (p. 74)

(Continued)

TABLE 4.2 (Continued)

REFERENCE	NUMBER OF PRESUMED CHILDREN WITH DAS REPORTED TO USE GESTURES AND VOCALIZATIONS	COMMENTS
Milloy & Summers, 1989	1/4	"Gesture: employed extensively to facilitate communication" (p. 297)
Hall, Hardy, & LaVelle, 1990	1/1	"Communicated by grunting and pointing, assisted by a form of 'sign language' " (p. 455)
Marquardt & Sussman, 1991	1/1	". . . attempted communication was accompanied by a well-developed gestural system" (p. 366)

We have followed a number of children with severe apraxic involvement who have developed fairly elaborate and individualized systems of gestures such as the child reported in Hall, Hardy, and LaVelle (1990). We have also seen children with DAS who use rudimentary formal signs. Clinicians are formalizing the young childrens' use of gestures so that the children are more easily understood by other than only specific family members, as is often the case with the development and use of idiosyncratic gestures. This issue will be more thoroughly explored in Chapter 9.

We have also found that children with DAS tend to use nonverbal mouth noises to assist in their communication attempts. Notable was one of our clients who successfully carried on a number of conversational turns about a cartoon character using only such mouth noises and gestures. While the use of these types of primitive methods of communication may be discouraging to parents and professionals alike, something positive must also be recognized—the child *is* attempting to communicate with others so communication must be important to them.

Assessment

While conducting a case history with the parent(s) of a child with suspected DAS, queries should be made into the possible development and use of gestural and nonverbal modes of communication and the success with which they are, or were, used. In addition, the clinician may wish to probe for characteristics of that child's verbal behavior that appear to be unique to that child such as a single utterance being used for many situations or meanings. The history may also reveal a developmental pattern that includes the loss of phonemes or words, which may be regained later.

Language Skills

The language skills of children with DAS addressed in the literature are reported in Table 4.3. Some references (Fawcus, 1971; Yoss & Darley, 1974a) either reported that the language skills were normal or included an essentially normal language function as a criterion for subject selection. However, the majority of references that include information regarding the language skills of children exhibiting DAS indicate that the children have difficulties with many domains of language, as well as with speech sounds (articulation or speech in the context of this text).

Some authors, particularly those writing in the early literature, described language abilities in the broad terms of receptive and expressive skills. The receptive skills were generally commented on, and found to be adequate, or at least further developed than the childrens' expressive skills (Aram & Glasson, 1979; Chappell, 1973; Eisenson, 1972; Lohr, 1978; McGinnis, 1963; Orton, 1937; Rapin & Allen, 1981; Riley, 1984; and Rosenbek & Wertz, 1972). However, the child with DAS may, in fact, have difficulties with the receptive aspects of language, although the expressive skills are much further depressed in relation to those involving comprehension and therefore demand more attention.

Gradually, with the evolution of thinking about developmental language disorders within the field, the various components of language were addressed in the literature concerning children with DAS. Syntax and semantics were the first such aspects to be observed or studied when Morley (1957) stated that some children with DAS she followed had problems in "use of words and sentence construction" (p. 228). Later authors also commented on problems in both semantic and syntactic comprehension and production. Snyder, Marquardt, and Peterson (1977) compared the results of the *Northwestern Syntax Screening Test* (Lee, 1971) that were administered to 30 boys; 10 subjects exhibited apraxia, 10 demonstrated functional articulation disorders, and 10 were developing language skills normally. Results indicated that the mean receptive scores achieved by the three subject groups were not significantly different. However, the mean expressive scores of the apraxic and functional articulation disordered groups were significantly reduced when compared to the normal boys, with the mean apraxic group scores lower than the mean achieved by the boys with functional articulation disorders.

TABLE 4.3
Descriptions of Language Skills of Children with DAS

REFERENCE	NUMBER OF CHILDREN WITH PRESUMED DAS EXHIBITING LANGUAGE DISORDERS REPORTED IN REFERENCE	DESCRIPTION OF LANGUAGE SKILLS
Orton, 1937	Not Reported	Children with "Developmental Motor Aphasia" had "good understanding of the spoken word" (p. 119)
Morley, 1957	NR/12	"In a few of the children there was an associated difficulty in the use of words and sentence construction, or developmental dysphasia, which continued into school and later life" (p. 228)
McGinnis, 1963	Not Reported	"Class I Motor Aphasia" characterized by "normal understanding of language" (p. 33)
Fawcus, 1971	Not Reported	"The true dyspraxic may have surprisingly normal language patterns" (p. 104)
Eisenson, 1972	Not Reported	"The child with 'congenital oral (articulatory) apraxia' does understand language" (p. 190)
Rosenbek & Wertz, 1972	28/50	"May occur . . . in combination with aphasia" "Receptive abilities are inordinately superior to expressive abilities" (p. 27)
Chappell, 1973	Not Reported	". . . expressive inadequacy contrasts remarkably with the essentially intact . . . receptive language performances of most of the children" (p. 362)
Yoss & Darley, 1974a	0/16	(For inclusion in the study the Language Age could be no more than 6 months below Chronologic Age)

(Continued)

TABLE 4.3 (Continued)

REFERENCE	NUMBER OF CHILDREN WITH PRESUMED DAS EXHIBITING LANGUAGE DISORDERS REPORTED IN REFERENCE	DESCRIPTION OF LANGUAGE SKILLS
Ferry, Hall, & Hicks, 1975	NR/60	(For inclusion in the study, the criteria of "normal or disproportionately high receptive language level" needed to be met)
Greene, 1967	Not Reported	". . . dyspraxia is always associated with language disorder. . . . telegraphic style . . . with paucity of vocabulary and immature syntax" (p. 19)
Snyder, Marquardt, & Peterson, 1977	10/10	"Children with developmental apraxia . . . do not demonstrate reduced knowledge of syntactical and morphonological rules . . . significantly reduced expressive grammatical skills observed for the apractic . . . group" (p. 153)
Lohr, 1978	5/5	All had expressive language limited to 3–30 words All had normal receptive language 3/5 were slightly below average in syntax comprehension
Aram & Glasson, 1979	8/8	Expressive vocabulary deficits Several subjects were anomic Syntactic formulation problems Comprehension of semantics and syntax often normal if nonverbal intelligence was normal, although length of sentences negatively affected comprehension

(Continued)

TABLE 4.3 (Continued)

REFERENCE	NUMBER OF CHILDREN WITH PRESUMED DAS EXHIBITING LANGUAGE DISORDERS REPORTED IN REFERENCE	DESCRIPTION OF LANGUAGE SKILLS
Rapin & Allen, 1981	Not Reported	"Hallmark of this ('phonologic programming deficit') syndrome is that comprehension is intact or at least good . . . discrepancy between adequate receptive skills and grossly deficient expression" (p. 33)
Ekelman & Aram, 1983, 1984	8/8	Expressive syntax deficits All subjects had problems with pronouns and primary verbs
Riley, 1984	8/15	Receptive-expressive gap of 1.5–3.0 standard deviations
Hall, Robin, & Jordan, 1986	5/5	Restricted receptive vocabularies Difficulties with word retrieval
Air, Wood, & Neils, 1989	Not Reported	Difficulties with "higher language processes of categorizing, organizing, and abstracting" (p. 273)
Milloy & Summers, 1989	4/4	Pragmatics Receptive skills syntax morphology vocabulary Expressive skills syntax morphology
Lucas, Weiss, & Hall, 1989, in press	3/3	Pragmatic difficulties in: Reduced informativeness Problems in adapting messages to reflect communicative demands placed on them

(Continued)

TABLE 4.3 (Continued)

REFERENCE	NUMBER OF CHILDREN WITH PRESUMED DAS EXHIBITING LANGUAGE DISORDERS REPORTED IN REFERENCE	DESCRIPTION OF LANGUAGE SKILLS
Adams, 1990	7/7	All thought by clinicians to have normal comprehension. Group mean on a comprehension task dealing with complex syntactical forms not significantly different from normal controls
Hall, Hardy, & LaVelle, 1990	1/1	Deficits in: Concept comprehension Expressive syntax Pragmatics Discourse Conversation management

Lohr (1978) noted that all five of the children with DAS she followed had expressive vocabularies of 3 to 30 words when they initially received clinical services as preschoolers. Three of the five children also had reduced comprehension of syntax. Adams (1990) assessed syntactic comprehension of seven children with "developmental dyspraxia," who ranged in ages from 4 years 7 months to 5 years 10 months. These four boys and three girls were given object manipulation and picture identification tasks involving the comprehension of the following complex syntactic stimuli: reversible active, embedded clauses, double object constructions, embedded phrases, and reversible passives. The performances of the dyspraxic children were compared to two groups of children of similar ages. One group had expressive language disorders and the second was a control group with normal language development. Results indicated that, in a syntactic decoding task, the group with dyspraxia and the control group performed similarly and without the subtle defects of comprehension displayed by children with defects of expressive syntax.

Aram and Glasson (1979) reported that the eight children with DAS they studied had deficits in expressive vocabulary and syntax. They also provide an excellent reminder that language skills must be evaluated within the context of any individual child's cognitive level. They found that comprehension of semantics and syntax was often normal when the nonverbal intelligence was normal. Notable among the listings contained in Table 4.3 are the references by Ekelman and Aram (1983, 1984). All eight of the subjects had deficits in use of pronouns and primary verbs. The readers are urged to refer to the original articles for detailed analyses of the children's specific syntactic deficits. Research we have conducted illustrates that restricted receptive vocabulary skills, as well as expressive syntax skills may be co-occurring symptoms in children with DAS (Hall, Robin, & Jordan, 1986; Hall, Hardy, & LaVelle, 1990).

Hall et al. (1990) commented that the subject of their case study (T.B.) had difficulties with pragmatics, specifically in the areas of discourse and conversation management. These deficit areas were targeted in the remedial program and were noted to improve over time. We recall that for several years T.B. developed and used single conversation starters such as "How you boys?" meaning, presumably, "How are your boys?" This initiator was used solely and singularly when T.B. wanted to start a conversation with one of us. While it was appropriate in some situations, such as once, or even twice a day, it was often inappropriate by its frequency—sometimes the requests were separated by as little as 45 minutes when she and the author saw each other both at the beginning and end of remedial sessions. Lucas, Weiss, and Hall (in press) also observed pragmatic differences in three children exhibiting DAS.

Problems may also be evidenced in the written language of children with DAS. We typically, to date, do not assess or develop remedial goals for this aspect of children's language. However, as a team member, we see this reflected in written work completed in the classroom with syntax being a particularly obvious deficit.

Air, Wood, and Neils (1989) stated that some children with DAS may not exhibit language problems until they enter the third or fourth grades. At that time problems in "higher language processes such as categorizing, organizing, and abstracting" (p. 273) may become evident. This should be kept in mind and justifies the monitoring of language skills in the child with DAS who, at younger ages, may exhibit normal (or nearly normal) language skills.

We have also noted word-retrieval problems within the language disorder of nearly all children presenting DAS we have followed. As reported in Hall, Robin, and Jordan (1986), we found that five children with DAS correctly identified fewer pictures in a confrontation naming task, identified the pictures more slowly, and exhibited more behaviors often associated with word- finding problems than did their age and sex-matched controls. Previously, Aram and Glasson (1979) had noted that several of their eight reported subjects with DAS were anomic. We have found that the word-retrieval problems of children demonstrating DAS are inconsistent as are their problems with speech sound production. For example, a second-grade boy on our caseload had great difficulties in accurately producing stops in multisyllabic words, despite consistent effort from session to session. During one session targeting two and three syllable words containing stops, he was very accurate with the articulatory goals but had great difficulties with word finding—a problem evidenced only rarely prior to that time. For him, "peacock" was initially "spike tail," then "colored tail," then "porcupine," and finally (with no clinician cuing), "peacock." During the particular session, this phenomenon was repeated on nearly every pictured stimulus item, but in following sessions the problem was again a rare occurrence.

Assessment

Language problems of varying severity have been evident in children with DAS who have been followed in our clinic. Many of our professional colleagues have remarked that they also have found this to be so with children diagnosed with developmental apraxia. Possibly this is because of increasing sophistication within the field in addressing the more subtle aspects of language disorders.

Formal and informal assessment procedures need to be used to gain an understanding and documentation of the language proficiency of children with DAS. As with any child exhibiting language disorders, the general level of the child's cognitive function must be kept in mind when results are interpreted. This, of course, assumes that intellectual appraisal is also included in early assessment procedures of a child with language disorders, including those who are suspected of exhibiting DAS.

We urge clinicians to evaluate semantic and syntactic comprehension early in their contact with children exhibiting DAS so that appropriate remedial goals can be set if necessary. We have found that it is often difficult to tease out what a child's expressive language competencies truly are due to lack of intelligibility of the expressive attempts. With some of the more severely involved children with DAS, we must be willing to wait until they are sufficiently intelligible to allow us to gain a picture of expressive language skills. With improved intelligibility, the speech-language professional can then be an accurate transcriber of expressive language, which can then be more formally analyzed along a number of parameters.

The presence of problems in the areas of pragmatic language use and word-retrieval problems have been noted in children with DAS. It is possible that many of the children with DAS, particularly those with severe limitations of intelligibility, have been denied early practice with discourse and interactive conversational skills. Thus, we urge early assessment of pragmatic skills as well, with appropriate remedial objectives put into effect where appropriate. Likewise, we often have found assessment of word-retrieval problems to be difficult due to the variability with which the problems are exhibited on a day-to-day basis. Thus, as suggested by Hall and Jordan (1987), assessment using a variety of methods, as well as observation over a period of time, might be the most effective way to document and describe word-finding problems in the language of children with DAS. If the problem is persistent, appropriate remedial goals should be developed to help the child learn self-cuing and compensatory strategies.

Presence of Academic Learning Problems

The academic prowess of children with developmental apraxia of speech needs to be examined because of the importance of literacy for survival in today's world and because of the importance much of society places on education itself. A summary of the relevant literature is presented in Table 4.4. As can be seen, several of the cited references (Morley 1957, 1959, 1965, 1972; Yoss & Darley, 1974a) found that only some of the children with developmental apraxia of speech had academic problems. Morley (1959) postulated that reading problems may be a developmental dyslexia "associated with articulatory apraxia" (p. 99). Yoss and Darley (1974a) concluded that learning difficulties "may or may not accompany" DAS (p. 413). The remaining references indicated that all children with DAS who were included in the studies also exhibited academic problems in the areas of reading, spelling, and mathematics.

The article by Snowling and Stackhouse (1983) is particularly interesting because it specifically addresses the spelling performances of four British children with *developmental verbal dyspraxia*. The children with dyspraxia and age-matched controls were given a general reading inventory in addition to specific experimental tasks consisting of imitation of verbal productions, spelling, reading, and copying CVC words. The children exhibiting dyspraxia were found to be comparable to their controls on the copying tasks but exhibited more problems than the controls with the imitation, spelling, and reading portions of the study. The children with dyspraxia also did poorer on these specific tasks than the results of the more general reading inventory had predicted. They made more errors on spelling than errors on the verbal imitation task, with more errors occurring on the final consonant than on the initial consonant. Other results of the study were that the children in the dyspraxia subject group had problems using a phonetic spelling strategy and were "less able to carry out grapheme-phoneme conversions than would be predicted from their reading ages" (p. 435). Further, the children with apraxia, whose scores on the standardized reading inventory matched the scores of their controls, were found to have more problems reading "simple, regular monosyllables" that were not a part of their sight vocabu-

TABLE 4.4
Review of Literature Addressing the Academic Skills of Children with DAS

REFERENCES	NUMBER OF CHILDREN WITH PRESUMED DAS REPORTED TO EXHIBIT ACADEMIC PROBLEMS	DESCRIPTIONS OF ACADEMIC PROBLEMS, WHEN PRESENT
Morley, 1957, 1959, 1965, 1972	4/12	Dyslexia (2 children) Spelling Disability (1 child) Dyslexia and Dysgraphia (1 child)
Yoss & Darley, 1974a	5/16*	"Received remedial help in special Learning Disability classes and were having difficulties in school achievement" (p. 412)
Mattis, French, & Rapin, 1975	14/14	"No child who had motor sequencing speech difficulty . . . was a fluent reader" (p. 154)
Greene, 1983	Not Reported	"Educational problems will arise" (p. 19)
Aram & Glasson, 1979	4/4	Reading Spelling Writing
Snowling & Stackhouse, 1983	4/4	Spelling Reading
Love & Fitzgerald, 1984	1/1	Spelling Reading
Milloy & Summers, 1989	4/4	Reading Spelling Writing
Hall, Hardy, & LaVelle (1990)	1/1	Reading Mathematics

*Also noted that an additional 5/16 subjects were "quite successful in their school work" (p. 412). (Recall that subject selection criteria included the requirement that language age could be no more than 6 months below chronological age.)

laries. These observations led Snowling and Stackhouse to suggest that it was inappropriate to rely greatly on phonic techniques in reading and spelling instruction with this group of students. Instead they suggested that instruction involve exposure to visual representations of words. Further descriptions of teaching strategies may be found in the original reference.

The possible occurrence of learning problems—most often reported to be in the form of reading and related skills—in children with DAS perhaps should not be surprising. Current thinking suggests that reading is a component of language, specifically within the phonological processing system (Catts, 1989). Many children with DAS exhibit language disorders. The problems children presenting DAS have within all language domains may also be reflected in their reading deficits. For instance, a child with a restricted vocabulary will likely have problems comprehending a written symbol when it represents a word or concept that they have not mastered. Syntax and morphology play important roles in both our written and spoken use of language; thus a child who does not understand or use a future tense verb or a past tense marker will also have difficulty fluently reading these forms with comprehension. Our observations suggest that word retrieval difficulties evidenced in the expressive language of many children with DAS are also evident in their attempts to retrieve written symbols during reading or writing. Moreover, problems with the production of phoneme sequences strikes at the heart of DAS and also may be reflected in the children's oral reading skills. Perhaps lack of experience in dealing with phoneme sequences at the production level may even be a factor in word analysis and breakdown in silent reading tasks.

As illustrated in the previous paragraphs, children presenting DAS, with their phonological sequencing difficulties and co-occurring language problems, are at risk in learning to read. It is unfortunate that much reading instruction is conducted as an expressive oral activity, which puts the child with DAS in severe instructional jeopardy.

School-age children with DAS whom we have followed seem to evidence academic problems. Some of the children's educational programming is conducted in self-contained Learning Disabilities or Communication Disordered classrooms, while others receive academic support through Resource Room assistance. Few, if any, of the children exhibiting DAS with whom we have had contact are prospering in the regular classroom without educational support programs other than speech and language services. However, we recognize that this observation may reflect the nature of the referrals to our clinic where the caseload tends to consist of the more severely involved individuals with communication disorders.

Assessment

We urge clinicians to be alert for the possible presence of academic problems with their clients demonstrating DAS. It is important to consult with the classroom teachers, suggest or make appropriate referrals to educational consultants, and share relevant information and observations with all members of the child's educational team. Furthermore, clinicians should also coordinate their remedial programming with the child's educational team members.

CHAPTER 5

Familial and Genetic Factors Associated with Children Exhibiting DAS

The areas to be addressed in this chapter include a number of familial and genetic factors that may be associated with DAS. Attempts to describe the population of individuals with DAS require that we address the presence of communication problems that are exhibited by other family members. We also need to acknowledge the presence of DAS in genetically-based syndromes and perhaps in specific inborn problems of metabolism. Further, an interesting issue to be discussed in this chapter is the numbers of boys versus girls with the problem.

Familial History

Children with DAS are often not alone in coping with their communication problems—many children find themselves in families where multiple other family members also experience, or have experienced, such problems. We are in agreement with Aram and Nation (1982) who stated: "We have been repeatedly impressed by both the frequency and the severity of other speech disorders in these children's families" (p. 164). Table 5.1 presents information from studies that report specific information on the family histories of children with DAS. The table summarizes the reported relationship of the family members to the child exhibiting DAS and the types of communication and learning problems reported to be present in the other family members.

Obviously we are still attempting to gain a better understanding of the etiological factors that contribute to the disorder. Although Horwitz (1984) concluded (in his study of the neurological findings of 10 children with *developmental verbal apraxia*) that the possible inheritance patterns did not represent a specific genetic factor, at least in some children there are suggestions of a genetic basis for developmental apraxia (Aram

TABLE 5.1
Review of Reported Family Histories of Children with DAS.

REFERENCE	NUMBER OF DAS CHILDREN WITH + HISTORY	RELATIVE(S) DEMONSTRATING COMMUNICATION AND/OR ACADEMIC PROBLEMS	TYPES OF COMMUNICATION AND EDUCATIONAL PROBLEMS REPORTED IN RELATIVES
Morley, 1957	6/12	Parents Grandfather Paternal uncle Sibling	Delayed speech development Stammer Articulation disorder
Ferry, Hall, & Hicks, 1975	17/60	Father Brother	Speech or Articulation problem
Aram & Glasson, 1979	5/8	Father Mother Identical twin Brother Paternal Grandmother Paternal aunt Maternal aunt Cousins	Delayed speech development Delayed articulation Reading & writing disorder Articulation disorder Stuttering Learning Disability
Horwitz, 1984	7/10	Mother Brother Twin Brother Maternal Uncle Paternal Cousin	Delayed speech Speech Language problem Reading problem

(Continued)

TABLE 5.1 (Continued)

REFERENCE	NUMBER OF DAS CHILDREN WITH + HISTORY	RELATIVE(S) DEMONSTRATING COMMUNICATION AND/OR ACADEMIC PROBLEMS	TYPES OF COMMUNICATION AND EDUCATIONAL PROBLEMS REPORTED IN RELATIVES
Crary, 1984a	Not reported	Fathers Paternal family members Occasional maternal family members	Delayed onset of speech Articulation problem Language development Stuttering Dyslexia
Riley, 1984	6/15	Not reported	Speech and/or language problems
Hall, 1989	1/1	Sister Paternal aunt Paternal uncle Maternal uncles Cousin	Articulation problems
Lewis, Ekelman, & Aram, 1989	4/5	Not reported	Included dyslexia
Milloy & Summers, 1989	3/4	S#1 Father Younger brother	S#1 "The same speech/language problems but to lesser degree" (p. 291)
		S#2 "Paternal side"	S#2 Stuttering Articulation disorder due to cleft palate

(Continued)

TABLE 5.1 (Continued)

REFERENCE	NUMBER OF DAS CHILDREN WITH + HISTORY	RELATIVE(S) DEMONSTRATING COMMUNICATION AND/OR ACADEMIC PROBLEMS	TYPES OF COMMUNICATION AND EDUCATIONAL PROBLEMS REPORTED IN RELATIVES
		S#3	S#3
		Unspecified	NR
Lewis, 1990	3/4	S#1	
		Brother	Phonological disorders
		Mother	Reading difficulties
		Maternal grandmother	
		Maternal uncle	
		Father	
		S#2	
		Brother	Articulation disorder
		Father	Dyslexia
		Paternal aunts	Stuttering
		Paternal uncle	Spelling difficulties
		Paternal grandmother	
		S#4	
		Brother	Apraxia
		Maternal uncles	Dyslexia
		Maternal female cousin	Speech problems
		Maternal male cousin	
		Father	
		Paternal grandfather	

& Glasson, 1979). A more recent pedigree analysis completed by Lewis, Ekelman, and Aram (1989) found a group of five pedigrees that were consistent with an autosomal dominant mode of inheritance, with four of the five probands having been diagnosed as exhibiting *verbal apraxia*. (In these genetic studies, a "proband" is the individual child exhibiting a particular trait on whom the selection of the entire family for study is based, and a "pedigree" is a description of the family members of a proband with respect to a particular trait.) All four probands were individuals with dyslexia. Lewis (1990) reported on four pedigrees which were traced through three generations and included three probands who exhibited apraxia. Although she stated that a genetic basis for severe phonological problems couldn't be conclusively demonstrated, her data supported a familial tendency that could be either genetically or environmentally based. Further, the four pedigrees were "consistent with either an autosomal dominant or multifactorial-polygenic mode of transmission with variable expressivity and penetrance" (p. 168). Lewis also noted that since all 4 probands were female, a sex-specific threshold for expression was suggested.

The works of Lewis (Lewis, Ekelman, & Aram, 1989; Lewis, 1990) have initiated much needed study into the genetics of families of children with DAS. Importantly, these studies have not relied solely on parental report for information. Professional evaluation of the academic and communication abilities of available family members are now beginning to define which relatives actually exhibit difficulties in these areas, as well as to define the nature and extent of the problems. Hopefully, larger numbers of pedigrees, spanning more generations of families, will be studied in the future. In addition, increasing sophistication in the study of genetics should enhance this area of investigation. Such studies have been conducted by Tomblin (1991).

Children with DAS with whom we have had contact often do come from families where numerous relatives also have communication difficulties. One such family is notable because through the years we have observed six family members from three generations. Our current client is severely apraxic; her older sister exhibited a speech sound disorder that included velopharyngeal difficulties. The client's preschool sister is being followed because of suspected delays in communication skills. The client has four aunts; her mother and one aunt were both childhood clients in our clinic. At the time they participated in our intensive residential program, both were diagnosed as presenting severe articulation and language problems. The client's mother continues to present language and articulation disorders that compromise intelligibility, and she has been observed during our interactions with her to present speech characteristics consistent with apraxia, most notably groping and silent posturing. A second aunt was also reported by the client's mother to have speech problems, although two other aunts did not. Interestingly, our present client's maternal grandmother was also observed by one of us to exhibit a severe articulation disorder that resulted in nearly unintelligible speech. The maternal grandfather presented no communication problems.

Assessment

We suggest that clinicians who have children with DAS on their caseloads attempt to obtain a good case history that includes information about the speech, language, and academic problems of all members of the child's immediate and extended family. Actually assessing these skills in the other family members, when possible, would also be helpful in better understanding which family members exhibit communication and academic problems and specifying the types of problems, the severity of the problems, and the actual impact on adult family members. Such information may be academic at the present time and not of help to the individual client. However, the accumulation of such information on larger groups of families may help us counsel future clients and their families by better defining if, and perhaps which, possible genetic factors may exist in the disorder of DAS.

Presence of DAS in Syndromes

Some family histories report the occurrence of DAS in individuals exhibiting established syndromes. Two of the subjects with *developmental verbal dyspraxia* studied by Ferry, Hall, and Hicks (1975) were reported to exhibit Down Syndrome, and one of Horwitz's (1984) 10 subjects with *developmental verbal apraxia* was reported to exhibit the chromosomal abnormality of an extra number 8 chromosome (trisomy 8). Two of this book's authors have followed a child with DAS who was diagnosed as exhibiting Robinow's Syndrome, an autosomal dominant genetic disorder involving multiple anomalies including craniofacial problems.

An emerging body of literature deals with fragile X syndrome. Jung (1989) states that this syndrome is genetically characterized by the occurrence of a fragile site on the long arm of the X chromosome at Xq27. Until recently, specialized cytogenetic techniques were required to demonstrate the presence of the fragile site. However, quicker, less expensive, and more reliable genetic tests are now available (Yu et al., 1991; Oberlé et al., 1991). Scharfenaker (1990) stated that fragile X is the most common heritable form of mental retardation. Because of the potential importance this syndrome may have in our work as speech-language pathologists, the topic will be covered in some detail. This will include statements about the presence of DAS as a component of the syndrome.

Early studies reported the presence of articulation and prosodic disorders as components of the fragile X Syndrome. For instance, Howard-

Peebles, Stoddard, and Mims (1979) reported seven of their 13 subjects "had difficulty with tongue control . . . it is possible that poor tongue control contributed to the articulation problems of this group." Turner, Daniel, and Frost (1980) and Jacobs et al., (1980) also noted speech disorders in their fragile X subjects.

Later reports indicated the specific presence of speech and oral apraxias as components of the syndrome. Newell, Sanborn, and Hagerman (1983) reported on 21 fragile X patients, all males ranging in age from 17 months to 31 years. An apraxia battery was included in their assessments. The presence of dyspraxia was noted in the spontaneous speech samples, which the article's authors indicated often lead to unintelligible speech. Imitation of polysyllabic words was said to be difficult for 100% of the subject group, and all subjects also had significant difficulty producing reduplicated consonant-vowel syllables (e.g., "pa-pa"), or trisyllable diadochokinetic patterns (e.g., "pa-ta-ka"). Newell, Sanborn, and Hagerman (1983) also reported other factors in the fragile X patients which we have noted as often co-occurring with DAS. For instance, all the Newell et al. patients had difficulty with volitional oral motor movements, particularly lateral tongue movements ("tongue wiggle"). Unusual prosodic and intonational patterns were documented during analysis of the spontaneous speech samples in 75% of their patients. While this was reported to be displayed most frequently in the latter half of utterances, Newell et al. also noted that in some cases a rising intonation pattern was observed in one-word utterances as well. Further, they noted that intonation patterns varied among the patients and were inconsistent within a single subject's speech. Receptive and expressive language deficits were described.

Paul, Cohen, Breg, Watson, and Herman (1984) reported on three individuals who presented fragile X syndrome. All three subjects exhibited speech characteristics consistent with DAS, including adequate production of speech sounds and words in isolation, with connected speech less intelligible than would be predicted on the basis of formal articulation testing; incorrect sequencing of a nonreduplicative syllable (/pʌtʌkʌ/); greater difficulty in production of multisyllabic words than was evidenced in bisyllabic words; and the presence of disfluencies consisting of prolongations and repetitions of sounds and syllables. Co-occurring language problems were suggested by receptive abilities that were superior to expressive skills.

Hanson, Jackson, and Hagerman (1986) evaluated 10 boys with fragile X syndrome who ranged in ages from 3 years 0 months to 8 years 10 months. They reported "severe apraxia was not seen in the imitation of single sounds and monosyllabic words. Mild to moderate motor planning problems were seen in all patients when polysyllabic words were imitated" (p. 201).

Madison, George, and Moeschler (1986) reported on 12 members (3 generations) of one family in which fragile X had been identified cytogenetically. The four affected adult males exhibited articulation errors of substitution and omissions, noted to usually occur with /r/-blends. One was noted to be difficult to understand when more than three words were spoken. All four were reported to evidence mild oral apraxia, with slow rate (less than half the normal mean) on diadochokinetic productions of single, bisyllabic, and trisyllabic repetitions. No oral or speech apraxia was noted in four of the five adult carrier females, although the rate for polysyllabic repetitions was more than one standard deviation below the adult mean. One woman exhibited a severe articulation disorder and mild oral and speech apraxia. Also of interest in this study was the description of hypernasality occurring in the nine adults presented. This included the four males and one female said to exhibit an oral or speech apraxia. Scharfenaker (1990) also listed the presence of "verbal dyspraxia" among the speech and language characteristics of males with fragile X.

Despite the current interest in fragile X, Jung (1989) noted that not all forms of X-linked mental retardation are associated with the fragile site, with some categorized as nonspecific X-linked mental retardation. For instance, McLaughlin and Kriegsmann (1980) reported on a family exhibiting Renpenning Syndrome, a syndrome with X-linked mental retardation but without physical abnormalities. *Developmental dyspraxia* was described as a prominent feature of this syndrome.

Assessment

Again, we suggest that clinicians attempt to obtain a good case history that includes information about any known genetic abnormalities within a client's immediate and extended family. Clinicians must also be alert for the presence of physical (morphologic) and behavioral features of various syndromes. There are references (Jung, 1989; Gorlin, Cohen, & Levin, 1990; McKusick, 1990) that can be helpful when syndromes are suspected. Such observations can result in referrals for genetic counseling, which may be necessary in diagnosing specific syndromes, and in helping families better understand their child and the implications of the genetic disorder.

Presence of DAS in Children with Inborn Errors of Metabolism

Nelson, Waggoner, Donnell, Tuerck, and Buist (1991) recently presented a study that revealed the presence of DAS in a group of children who had been treated for galactosemia. This is an autosomal, recessively inherited inborn error of metabolism with the incidence of approximately 1:60,000 children born in the United States. A milk enzyme crucial to the conversion of galactose to glucose is deficient in patients presenting this problem.

Nelson et al. reported on 24 children who had been treated for galactosemia. Thirteen of the subjects, representing 54% of those studied, were found to exhibit *verbal dyspraxia*. Of these subjects, one was rated as having a mild problem, although she was a high school student at the time of the project and had a history of a severe speech disorder as a child. She was reported to have received extensive remediation services. Six of the subjects were rated as presenting a moderate dyspraxia, and the other six were rated as presenting a severe dyspraxia. In addition to the speech characteristics associated with DAS, the 13 apraxic subjects were also found to have problems with syntax and word-retrieval in the language domain.

The Nelson et al. study further revealed that the presence or severity of the verbal dyspraxia was *not* related to a variety of factors such as: (1) the age at which dietary modifications were initiated, (2) the compliance to the diet at the time of testing, (3) the severity of the medical symptoms associated with the galactosemia in the subjects during the neonatal period, (4) the age at which diagnosis of the condition was made, and (5) gender.

Interestingly, Nelson et al. found that two additional subjects presented non-apraxic developmental or functional articulation problems. Thus, 15 of the 24 subjects presented some type of speech sound disorder.

The study concluded that even those infants with classic galactosemia who were identified at birth and received rigorous dietary treatment are at risk for long-term difficulties. Included in the potential problems encountered later in life may be speech sound disorders. The data from Nelson et al. indicate that the risk for DAS may be particularly high in this population.

Assessment

The results of the Nelson, Waggoner, Donnell, Tuerck, and Buist (1991) study present a caution to speech-language pathologists. As professionals we need to be aware of clients and patients who have a history of at least this one type of metabolic disorder. This will mean that we need to probe into dietary issues within case histories and work with physicians and dieticians who are primary medical team members working with a particular child. As well, we need to be cognizant of this new information and explore the possibilities of the unreported presence of DAS in children with other types of metabolic disorders.

Sex Ratios

The literature is replete with reports that DAS is more likely to occur in boys than girls, although it is not thought to be an exclusively male disorder. This issue has been discussed by Aram and Nation (1982) and Crary (1984a). Table 5.2 presents the number and percentages of boys and girls with DAS, in the present body of literature, when gender information has been provided. Table 5.3 indicates the gender of the single-subject case studies that have also been reported.

TABLE 5.2
Reported Sex Ratios of Children Exhibiting DAS

REFERENCE	TOTAL NUMBER REPORTED CHILDREN WITH DAS	NUMBER (%) MALES WITH DAS		NUMBER (%) FEMALES WITH DAS	
Hadden, 1891	2	2	(100%)	0	(0%)
Morley, 1957, 1959, 1965, 1972	12	7	(58%)	5	(42%)
Rosenbek & Wertz, 1972	50	38	(76%)	12	(24%)
Ferry, Hall, & Hicks, 1975	60	40	(67%)	20	(33%)
Aram & Glasson, 1979	8	8	(100%)	0	(0%)
McLaughlin & Kriegsmann, 1980	2	2	(100%)	0	(0%)
Krauss & Galloway, 1982	2	2	(100%)	0	(0%)
Towne & Crary, 1982	8	7	(88%)	1	(12%)
Ekelman & Aram, 1983	8	7	(88%)	1	(12%)
Bowman, Parsons, & Morris, 1984	7	7	(100%)	0	(0%)
Crary, Landess, & Towne, 1984	10	8	(80%)	2	(20%)
Ekelman & Aram, 1984	3	2	(67%)	1	(33%)
Horwitz, 1984	10	8	(80%)	2	(20%)
Parsons, 1984	7	6	(86%)	1	(14%)
Schumacher, McNeil, Vetter & Yoder, 1984	3	2	(67%)	1	(33%)
Hall, Robin, & Jordan, 1986	5	3	(60%)	2	(40%)
LaVoi, 1986	20	16	(80%)	4	(20%)
Robin, Hall, & Jordan, 1986, 1987	5	3	(60%)	2	(40%)
Jackson & Hall, 1987	4	2	(50%)	2	(50%)
Milloy & Summers, 1989	4	2	(50%)	2	(50%)
Pollock & Hall, 1989, 1991	5	4	(80%)	1	(20%)
Lewis, 1990	4	0	(0%)	4	(100%)
Betsworth & Hall, 1989	5	3	(60%)	2	(40%)
Robin, Hall, Jordan, & Gordan, 1991	3	2	(67%)	1	(33%)

TABLE 5.3
Sex of Children with DAS Reported in Single-Subject Case Studies

REFERENCE	MALE WITH DAS	FEMALE WITH DAS
Dabul, 1971	1	—
Rosenbek, Hansen, Baughman, & Lemme, 1974	—	1
Doszak, McNeil, & Jancosek, 1981	1	—
Harlan, 1984	1	—
Davis, Marquardt, & Sussman, 1985	1	—
Klick, 1985	—	1
Shelton & Graves, 1985	1	—
Goldwasser, 1989	—	1
Hall, 1989	—	1
Hall, Hardy, & LaVelle, 1990	—	1
Marquardt & Sussman, 1991	1	—

Generally, boys are represented in the literature in greater numbers than girls. Crary (1984a) stated that "approximately 80-90% of our subjects are male" (pp. 36-37). However, the male-female ratio varies from study to study. Further, it must be noted that in some studies, the sexes were equally represented as is reflected in the nine case studies reviewed on Table 5.3. Of the total population of children with DAS reported in the literature, excluding our research (Tables 5.2 and 5.3), 74% (170 of 229 total) are males.

Data from a study by Lewis (1990) is particularly interesting in that she reported her four probands with severe phonological disorders were all female. She noted that this finding was contrary to typical sex ratios for children with phonologic disorders; three of these girls had been diagnosed as verbally apractic and the fourth presented many characteristics consistent with this diagnosis.

In our diagnostic clinic, we see nearly equal numbers of girls and boys with DAS. This may reflect the nature of the referrals to our clinic, which is a tertiary level facility serving an entire state. Thus, the referrals we receive may be skewed so that we see a greater proportion of severely disordered children than may be present in the typical caseload. Nonetheless, we noted with some interest that the sex ratios reflected in our own research reveal a different trend than that typically reflected in the literature. In fact, only 50% (6 of 12 total) of the DAS subjects participating in our studies were males; a number of our subjects have been involved in several of our projects.

We find several observations relating to the sex ratios exhibited in the population of children with DAS to be of interest: (1) our experience of equal numbers of referrals for girls with DAS as for boys with DAS, (2) that usually both the boys and girls seen by us exhibit severe DAS, and (3) the all-female study presented by Lewis (1990). These observations may reflect the "threshold model" for the expression of DAS in females. Using this concept from genetics, a condition, such as DAS, that seems to exhibit prevalence rates according to sex will be expressed when a particular threshold is crossed. For DAS this may mean that a higher threshold, with greater loading of factors, is necessary before a female exhibits the disorder. However, greater loading may result in the disorder being exhibited in a more severe form. Perhaps there are fewer females with DAS, but it may be that when DAS does occur, they are severely disordered.

CHAPTER 6

Neurologic and Psychologic Factors: Co-occurring Characteristics of Children Exhibiting DAS

The previous two chapters have discussed characteristics and associated findings that may be evident in children presenting DAS.
While perhaps not central to the speech problems they are exhibiting, these factors are observed with enough frequency that we think they
may co-occur with the problem of DAS. These children often bring still
other associated problems with them, which fall into the neurological
and psychological areas and which must be accounted for when speech-
language pathologists are looking at the "total" child. Thus, this chapter
will address findings suggestive of possible or definitive neurological
involvement, oral mechanism (nonverbal) function problems, auditory
perceptual deficits, as well as intelligence, personality, and behavior. As
we begin assessment and treatment programs, our sensitivity to these
related problems increases. As with the preceding chapters, we will share
our current thinking regarding the impact of each factor on management
issues. It is our intention to share suggestions on assessment techniques
as they relate to these accompanying characteristics which children with
DAS may demonstrate.

Findings Suggestive of Neurological Involvement

Any discussion of developmental apraxia of speech eventually turns to
the question of whether these children have a discrete lesion in the nervous system. This question seems particularly relevant in that the parents of children with DAS and some clinicians assume that there is a well
defined neurological abnormality. Some of these parents may have
received this suggestion from the referring clinician or physician, while
others have received the information from other sources. An assumption
of "brain damage" exists because much of what is theorized about DAS
stems from comparisons of DAS with acquired apraxia of speech in adults.

Children with DAS are often described by parents and practitioners as being clumsy and uncoordinated. Their histories often indicate late achievement of motor milestones. The literature also seems to suggest these trends (see Table 6.1), although few studies have systematically investigated such aspects of children with DAS.

The interest in whether DAS is neurologically based is twofold. First, if there is a well defined anatomical lesion that consistently produces DAS, it would affect the referrals we make as well as our treatment of these clients. If not, we can rule out the presence of the onus of "brain damage." However, it may be helpful to look at the profile of behaviors that is assumed to represent neurological soft signs and to examine other potential explanatory mechanisms. A second reason to be interested in the neurological observations is that they may offer potential explanation about the neural substrates and the developmental progression of speech motor control.

In recent years technological advances have allowed for the examination of the brain, in vivo, via such techniques as electroencephalography (EEG), computerized tomographic (CT) scans, magnetic resonance imaging (MRI), single photon emission computed tomography (SPECT), and positron emission tomography (PET). The existing literature is small and the findings of investigations with children exhibiting DAS are mixed (see Table 6.2) as to the presence or absence of significant anatomical differences and/or lesions as well as the critical location(s). The CT scans of children with DAS seem to have produced more evidence of abnormalities than have the EEG techniques used to date. Nonetheless, there are reports of normal CT scans in children with DAS.

Aram and Glasson (1979) reported that five of their eight children with *developmental verbal apraxia* had undergone EEGs, and all five were normal. Six of the eight had received CT scans; four were normal, while one scan had posterior abnormalities (expansion of quadrigeminal cistern and prominence of vermin cistern), and one scan revealed questionable bilateral parietal-occipital-temporal atrophy. Horwitz (1984) studied 10 children with *developmental verbal apraxia.* Of the nine who had CT scans, seven were normal. The two abnormal scans were dissimilar but involved the ventricular system and not neuronal tissue. In other words, these studies showed no consistent neurologic involvement across subjects as well as no evidence of focal lesions.

Denays et al. (1989) presented data on 14 French-speaking children with congenital dysphasia, two of whom were described as having *verbal dyspraxia.* EEGs and CT scans were normal for all children involved in the study. The children, including the two with dyspraxia, also underwent SPECT study, a procedure that documents cerebral blood flow. Only symmetric differences of greater than 12% between regions of the brain were considered significant. Both dyspraxic children were found to demonstrate hypoperfusion in the inferior frontal convolutions of the left hemisphere involving Broca's area.

TABLE 6.1

Reports of Neurological Findings (Through Clinical Examination,
Clinical Observation, and History) in Children with DAS

REFERENCE	NUMBER OF CHILDREN WITH PRESUMED DAS INCLUDED IN REPORT	COMMENT
Hadden, 1891	1	"He was left handed for all purposes, although he could use his right hand as well, or nearly as well, as his left . . . . He could write with both the right and the left hand" (pp. 96, 98).
Orton, 1937	1	late in developing a preference for either right or left hand.
		case description of 12-year-old: slow in learning to walk awkward in gait unable to ride bicycle roller skate play baseball no hand preference unacceptable penmanship
Morley, 1957	67	61% were right handed 20% were ambidextrous for eye, hand, or foot 49% showed cross-laterality "highly significant number of children with absence of dominant gradient" (p. 399)
Walton, Ellis, & Court, 1962	3	subject VP—12 years old: walked at 2 years of age clumsy in dressing clumsy in handling objects and tools extremely poor writing unable to handle cricket bat and ball could not jump over lowest obstacle left handed and eyed kicked a ball with either foot muscular activity clumsy, slow, and "ill-directed" (p. 605)

(Continued)

TABLE 6.1 (Continued)

REFERENCE	NUMBER OF CHILDREN WITH PRESUMED DAS INCLUDED IN REPORT	COMMENT

		subject DL—12 years old:
		  unable to make hands "perform necessary actions" (p. 605)
		  clumsy gait and movements of limbs
		  right handed, right eyed, left footed
		  "crude" handwriting (p. 605)
		subject DN—9 years old:
		  clumsy use of limbs
		  unable to dress or handle eating utensils
		  poor writing and drawing
		  unable to throw or catch a ball
		  apraxia of tongue and lips
		  "used both hands, but probably preferred the right. A ball was kicked equally often with the two feet" (p. 606)

Gubbay, Ellis, Walton, & Court, 1965	5	5 subjects with "articulatory apraxia" were included in subject group of 14 who exhibited "severe clumsiness" and isolated apraxia and agnosia. Descriptions of associated behaviors are listed (p. 304), but not by subject. "poor writing, which was almost universal, was probably largely a function of associated contructional apraxia" (p. 305) "one of the remarkable features of the syndrome is the practically universal 'fidgetiness' that is exhibited" (p. 310)
Eisenson, 1972	Not Reported	"histories . . . suggest some degree of overall dyspraxia. Some children are conspicuously awkward, early developmental histories include late walking and severe lack of manual dexterity. Handedness and other indications of laterality preference may not be established by age five . . .

(Continued)

TABLE 6.1   (Continued)

REFERENCE	NUMBER OF CHILDREN WITH PRESUMED DAS INCLUDED IN REPORT	COMMENT
		ambi-nonlateral, slow, and awkward in all forms of motor expression" (p. 195)
Rosenbek & Wertz, 1972	50	36/50 had neurological examinations 22/36 "essentially normal" *except*: 12/22—oral apraxia 7/22—orofacial apraxia 3/22—unspecified apraxia 14/36 had neurological deficits: 8/14—hyperreflexia and spasticity 3/14—muscle weakness 2/14—hyperkinesia 1/14—hyperreflexia and muscle weakness 11/50 were reported to have excessive drooling "DAS may occur in isolation or in combination with aphasia or dysarthria" (p. 27) 9/50—DAS alone 20/50—DAS and aphasia 13/50—DAS and dysarthria 8/50—DAS, aphasia, and dysarthria
Yoss & Darley, 1974a	16	15/16 had positive neurological findings decreased alternate motion rate of the tongue and extremities difficulties in gait and coordination history of difficulties: manipulating scissors, buttons, zippers tying shoelaces fell often awkward in playground activities ". . . high incidence of 'soft' neuro- logic findings . . . often manifested as a generalized dyspraxia" (p. 413)

(Continued)

TABLE 6.1   (Continued)

REFERENCE	NUMBER OF CHILDREN WITH PRESUMED DAS INCLUDED IN REPORT	COMMENT
Ferry, Hall, & Hicks, 1975	60	all had neurological examinations: 36/60—orofacial dyspraxia 13/60—mild spastic diplegia 10/60—mild motor retardation 2/60—hand tremor 2/60—Down Syndrome 1/60—hemiplegia 1/60—choreiform movements "high percentage" of subjects had associated signs of oral or facial dyspraxia ". . . persistent and excessive drooling and difficulty with chewing, licking and sucking movements" (p. 751)
Lohr, 1978	5	4/5 had generalized body apraxia no histories of feeding problems
Aram & Glasson, 1979	8	7 had neurological examinations 2/7—normal 3/7—idiosyncratic positive findings 6/7—difficulties standing and hopping on one foot, and skipping 3/7—difficulties with coordinating alternating hand movements 2/7—right hand preference 0/7—left hand preference 5/7—mixed or questionable hand preference
Aram & Horwitz, 1981	10	"As a group," the children with "developmental verbal apraxia" did not have deficits on tasks of manual gestures and constructional abilities, although, variations were present among the subjects
Kornse, Manni, Rubenstein, & Graziani, 1981	18	no differences between performances in right and left hand manual dexterity tasks in both male and female subjects

(Continued)

TABLE 6.1 (Continued)

REFERENCE	NUMBER OF CHILDREN WITH PRESUMED DAS INCLUDED IN REPORT	COMMENT
		all female DAS subjects (9) had impaired manual dexterity of both hands, while no male DAS subject (9) had such impairment, when compared to normal controls
Williams, Ingham, & Rosenthal, 1981	15	1/15 subjects was reported to have a positive neurological finding
Aram & Nation, 1982	Not Reported	". . . neurologic findings with developmentally apraxic children are equivocal at best" (p. 161)
Darwish, Pearce, Gaines, & Harasym, 1982	10	7/10 had abnormal neurological findings 2/7 subjects with "speech programming deficit syndrome" had mild hemiparesis 6/7 had difficulties imitating facial and lingual movements
Crary, 1984a	25	evidence or history of "motor clumsiness" used as a criteria for selection in "Developmental Verbal Dyspraxic" subject group *none had evidence of motor weakness *"many" subjects had direct or reported fine motor incoordination *file reviews: 13/25—motor incoordination 1/25—mild spasticity 6/25—no obvious problems (*see page 36)
Horwitz, 1984	10	all had neurological examinations 2/10—no abnormal neurological findings 8/10—had neurological abnormalities 5/10—late in walking 5/10—ocular abnormalities

(Continued)

TABLE 6.1 (Continued)

REFERENCE	NUMBER OF CHILDREN WITH PRESUMED DAS INCLUDED IN REPORT	COMMENT
		4/5—esotropia
		1/5—incomplete third nerve paralysis
		2/10—increased deep tendon reflexes
		1/10—macrencephaly
		1/10—oral apraxia
		1/10—limb apraxia
		1/10—gait ataxia
		1/10—hypotonia with hyperextensible joints
		1/10—bilateral Babinski sign
		1/10—severe synkinesis and spasticity of heel cords
		1/10—clumsy, awkward gait
Riley, 1984	15 had severe syllable production problems *plus* a minimum of 6/11 DVD symptoms	5/15 (33%) had attention and/or impulsivity problems
Wiznitzer, Rapin, & Allen, 1986	6	all 6 subjects with "verbal dyspraxia" had abnormalities of gross and/or fine motor function, especially in tasks involving alternating movement or rate of movement
		1/6 subjects had mild hemiparesis with contralateral handedness and bilateral motor dysfunction
		"verbal dyspraxic" children were more likely to have fine motor and visumotor scores below the 10th percentile on the *Purdue Pegboard Test* than were children with other types of developmental language disorders
		oromotor dysfunction also occurred more frequently with the "verbal dyspraxia" group

(Continued)

TABLE 6.1 (Continued)

REFERENCE	NUMBER OF CHILDREN WITH PRESUMED DAS INCLUDED IN REPORT	COMMENT
Hall, Hardy, & LaVelle, 1990	1	parents described client as "clumsy" "fine motor incoordination" was diagnosed by pediatric neurologist nystagmus

Recently, using MRI techniques, we studied the brains of three children with a diagnosis of severe DAS (unpublished data). There was no evidence of focal lesions in any of the children studied, although one scan suggested a possible developmental anatomical difference in the left frontal operculum.

With the interest in questions regarding the potential neurological substrates involved in DAS have come hypotheses about the neurological origins of the disorder. These are summarized on Table 6.3 and reflect diverse opinions.

We often describe children exhibiting DAS as displaying clumsiness and a lack of coordination in their motor behaviors. It appears as if some of the children with DAS can be described as being unable to simultaneously walk and talk; seeming to be unable to maintain motor control over two systems at the same time. Yet, we also have observed children with DAS who exhibit minimal, if any, motor involvement other than that demonstrated during oral movements and in their speech attempts.

While we think that neurological examinations may be potentially helpful in gaining a better understanding of an individual child with DAS as well as helpful in advancing general knowledge about the disorder, it is difficult to routinely obtain such information. Medical examinations of this type are typically expensive and are often difficult to justify on this basis alone, particularly for those children about whom we have no specific neurological questions.

The neurological status of children with DAS is an interesting and necessary aspect of investigation. Perhaps as future technologies are developed and refined more answers (and questions) will be forthcoming.

Presence/Absence of Nonspeech Oral Apraxia

Love (1992) defines *developmental oral apraxia* as an "apraxia of nonspeech acts," in that it is an "inability to perform voluntary movements

TABLE 6.2
Reports of Laboratory Findings in Children with DAS

REFERENCE	NUMBER OF CHILDREN WITH PRESUMED DAS INCLUDED IN REPORT	COMMENT
Rosenbek & Wertz, 1972	50	26/50 had EEGs 11/26—normal 10/26—generalized cortical disturbances without lateralizing or localizing significance 5/26—focal abnormalities 2/5—focal bilateral abnormalities involving the motor strip (1), and the Sylvian and parietal regions (1) 3/5—disruption confined to right hemisphere, with a temporal-parietal lobe lesion (1), temporal lobe and reduced activity (1), and a right parietal and posterior temporal foci (1) suggested
Ferry, Hall, Hicks, 1975	60	20 subjects, residents of a state institution for persons with mental retardation, had EEGs. All were "mildly and non specifically abnormal with mild, generalized slowing and occasional sharp wave activity. No localized abnormalities were seen" (p. 751)
Aram & Glasson, 1979	8	5/5—normal EEGs 4/6—normal CT scans 1/6—possible bilateral parietal-occipital temporal atrophy 1/6—posterior expansion of quadrigeminal cistern and prominence of vermin cistern
Darwish, Pearce, Gaines, & Harasym, 1982	10	4/10 with "speech programming deficit syndrome" had small, atrophic, lateralized lesions on CT scans 2/4—to right 2/4—to left

(Continued)

TABLE 6.2 (Continued)

REFERENCE	NUMBER OF CHILDREN WITH PRESUMED DAS INCLUDED IN REPORT	COMMENT

Horwitz, 1984	10	9/9—normal EEGs
		7/9—normal CT scans
		2/9—abnormal CT scans
		   1/2—enlarged cisterns around cerebellum and lower brain stem
		   1/2—enlarged occipital horns
		7/7—normal urine amino acid chromatography

Denays, Tondeur, Foulon, Verstraeten, Ham, Piepsz, & Noel, 1989	2	2/2—normal EEGs 2/2—normal CT scans 2/2—SPECT study-hypoperfusion in inferior frontal convolution of left hemisphere, involving Broca's area

of the muscles of the pharynx, tongue, cheeks, and lips, although automatic movements of these muscles may be preserved'' (p. 10). As is obvious from the review below, the literature on the presence of oral apraxia in DAS is controversial. However, the motor control for speech requires an extremely high level of coordination and precision, both within and between individual speech articulators and other speech production systems. The finding that some children with DAS do not have difficulty with the relatively simple oral movements typically tested in the clinic (e.g., stick out your tongue, smile and then pucker) does not imply that oral apraxia does not exist. Robin (1992) has argued that if an oral apraxia for relatively simple movements exists, then an apraxia for speech also will be present. He goes on to note that clinicians may need to consider using more complex tests for oral motor control before deciding that apraxia for nonspeech purposes is absent.

Information from the literature concerning the co-existence of oral apraxia and developmental apraxia of speech is presented in Table 6.4. As with many of the other factors discussed in this chapter, there is not a consensus regarding the co-occurrence of oral apraxia and DAS. An early Morley reference (1957) stated there was not a problem with this form of apraxia with DAS, although in a 1959 reference, she modified this

TABLE 6.3
Descriptions of Hypothesized Neurological Origins of DAS

REFERENCES	NUMBER OF CHILDREN WITH PRESUMED DAS INCLUDED IN REPORT	COMMENTS
Gubbay, Ellis, Walton, & Court, 1965	5	(articulatory apraxia) . . . "is presumed to be a disturbance of function arising at a higher level in the effector pathways of speech in the nervous systems than in a patient with facial and lingual apraxia" (p. 305)
Luchsinger & Arnold, 1965	Not Reported	"dyspractic articulation reflects a basic disorder of neural-muscular balance" (p. 383)
Morley & Fox, 1969	Not Reported	"articulatory dyspraxia is considered to be due to a disturbance of function arising in the sensorimotor pathways for speech in the nervous system" (p. 157)
Rosenbek & Wertz, 1972	50	"suggested . . . praxis centers for speech movements in the child's cortex may be quite diffuse" (p. 25) "It may be that young children have large areas in both hemispheres essential to the development of volitional, skilled performance. At some point praxis centers for skilled movement may lateralize, usually to the left hemisphere, and become more discretely localized. Before such lateralization and localization take place, any of a variety of left-right, anterior-posterior lesions may result in apraxia of speech" (p. 26)
Ferry, Hall, & Hicks, 1975	60	"Since no autopsy studies have been performed, the exact basis of this puzzling, highly selective speech disorder remains elusive" (p. 753)

(Continued)

TABLE 6.3 (Continued)

REFERENCES	NUMBER OF CHILDREN WITH PRESUMED DAS INCLUDED IN REPORT	COMMENTS
Aram & Nation, 1982	8	". . . these children demonstrated very little evidence for focal cortical problems, and in particular not for anteriorly placed cortical lesions" (p. 162)
Chumpelik, 1984	Not Reported	". . . typically no specific lesion sites are recognizable . . . Diffuse damage in which possible 'mini-lesions' or subtle 'wiring' difficulties exist, may be more the case" (p. 140)
Crary, 1984a	25	Children with "developmental verbal dyspraxia possess a selective neurolinguistic deficit in the left hemisphere phonological component of the perisylvian central language system" (p. 45)
Horwitz, 1984	10	study "failed to demonstrate consistent neurological findings or a specific localizing anatomical basis for clinical manifestations of DVA . . . neurological abnormalities are quite varied with no consistent patterns . . . it is evident that neurological findings in children with DVA are diverse and that the underlying nervous system abnormalities remain undefined. . . . It is improbable that an isolated biochemical or neurotransmitter is causative" (pp. 116–117)
Wiznitzer, Rapin, & Allen, 1986	6	"increased prebalance of oromotor and fine motor dysfunction in children with expressive deficits (verbal dyspraxia) compared to those with disorders of semantic comprehension and formation suggests more anterior pathology in the former" (pp. 413–414)

(Continued)

TABLE 6.3   (Continued)

REFERENCES	NUMBER OF CHILDREN WITH PRESUMED DAS INCLUDED IN REPORT	COMMENTS
Thompson, 1988	Not Reported	etiology of DAS is unknown
Denays, Tondeur, Foulon, Verstraeten, Ham, Piepsz, & Noel, 1989	2	"the hypofixation found in the Broca's area could explain the expression impairments in the two patients with verbal dyspraxia" (p. 1828)
Love, 1992	Not Reported	"It is assumed lesions are at higher levels of the nervous system" (p. 11). ". . . as yet neurological research has not associated Broca's area with DVD" (p. 43)

stand, stating that nonspeech movements *may* be within the normal range. References since that time generally take the posture that oral apraxia may, or may not, accompany DAS.

The diagnosis of oral apraxia in Rosenbek and Wertz's study (1972) was made during pediatric neurological examinations conducted by physicians. Thirty-six children received this type of examination; 12 were found to have a generalized apraxia including an oral apraxia, and seven were found to exhibit an apraxia confined to orofacial musculature. Horwitz (1984), a pediatric neurologist, also diagnosed one child within his 10 subjects as having an oral apraxia during a pediatric neurological physical examination.

We realize that an oral apraxia may not necessarily be evident in a child with DAS depending on how oral movement control is tested. However, our experience has been that the two factors have co-existed in all children exhibiting DAS we have followed to date. We acknowledge that this observation may be colored by the severely disordered children with DAS who are referred to us and by the sensitivity of our assessment procedures. Perhaps children with severe DAS may be the ones most at risk for, and most likely to exhibit, oral apraxia. Thus, we have not yet seen a child with what some would call a *pure* DAS, with no evidence of an oral apraxia also being present. However, such a child may walk through our clinic doors tomorrow.

TABLE 6.4

Presence or Absence of an Accompanying Oral (Facial) Apraxia

REFERENCE	NUMBER OF CHILDREN WITH PRESUMED DAS	DESCRIPTION
Morley, 1957	12	". . . there was no limitation of movement of lips, tongue, or palate, and such movement appeared normal when carried out voluntarily on request" (p. 227)
Morley, 1959	Not Reported	". . . spontaneous, involuntary imitation of movements of the tongue or lips on request may be within the normal range" (p. 94)
Morley & Fox, 1969	Not Reported	"articulatory dyspraxia . . . can result from an oral dyspraxia, it would seem to occur when no oral disability can be detected" (p. 157)
Eisenson, 1972	Not Reported	"the child is impaired in executing movements with specific parts of the oral mechanism . . . difficulties tend to increase if rapid movement is expected or a series of movements are required" (pp. 192–193)
Rosenbek & Wertz, 1972	50	oral apraxia often accompanies DAS, but "apraxia of speech may occur in isolation" (p. 26)
Yoss & Darley, 1974a	16	an accompanying oral apraxia is usually apparent had difficulty with isolated and sequential volitional oral movements, especially with movements involving the tongue and lips required more demonstrations to perform sequences of volitional oral movements
Ferry, Hall, & Hicks, 1975	60	36/60 had signs of associated oral and/or facial dyspraxia
Lohr, 1978	5	all demonstrated normal vegetative function of the oral structures
Rapin & Wilson, 1978	Not Reported	some children may have oral-motor apraxia

(Continued)

TABLE 6.4 (Continued)

REFERENCE	NUMBER OF CHILDREN WITH PRESUMED DAS	DESCRIPTION
Aram & Glasson, 1979	8	"a nonspeech oral apraxia may, but does not necessarily, accompany verbal apraxia" (p. 163) 4/8 had difficulty producing single nonspeech movements 5/8 had difficulty producing a sequence of nonspeech volitional movements
Aram & Horwitz, 1981	10	children with "developmental verbal apraxia" as a group, had difficulties with sequential nonverbal volitional oral movements
Horwitz, 1984	10	1/10 demonstrated oral apraxia during neurological examination
Love & Fitzgerald, 1984	1	difficulty with: elevated and lateral tongue movements, rate, accuracy and strength nonspeech oral apraxia appeared to resolve during later evaluation
Murdoch, Porter, Younger, & Ozanne, 1984	Not Applicable	inability to achieve isolated and sequenced oral movements on command was one of three characteristics identified by 30 Australian clinicians as consistently associated with DVD
Riley, 1984	15	9/15 (60%) presented moderate to severe nonverbal oral-motor problems
Hall, 1989	1	difficulty performing nonspeech single and sequenced volitional oral movements, with errored or omitted movements being exhibited
Hall, Hardy, & LaVelle, 1990	1	sequences of nonspeech oral movements were difficult, with slowed rates and imprecision of movement patterns
Love, 1992	Not Reported	"developmental oral apraxia may or may not accompany DVD" (p. 16)

Can oral apraxia disappear? Love and Fitzgerald's 1984 case study reports that the child's nonspeech oral apraxia had resolved during the third evaluation conducted through their clinic. Over 5 years had elapsed between the initial evaluation (when the child was reported to be unable to elevate or lateralize the tongue) and the evaluation (when adequate strength and movement of the articulators was noted). At that time the child was 7 years 9 months of age. Generally, resolution of oral apraxia has not been evident with the children exhibiting DAS followed through our clinic. While many of the children we have followed continue to have problems with non-speech movements, they show decreased problems with such movements over time. However the problems have not totally resolved. Again, the severity of the total set of disorders exhibited by the children with DAS known to us may be influencing this observation. We may also be influenced by our stringent assessment procedures which may stress the child's ability to produce non-speech, as well as speech movements to such a degree that we are less accepting than those professionals with a more modest examination might be.

We have often observed that the tasks used to test for oral apraxia may be too simple. Thus, we advocate the development and use of tasks that stress the oral motor control capabilities in a similar manner as speech may shed light on the presence of oral apraxia as well as eventually point to new treatment techniques.

Assessment

The functional adequacy of the oral peripheral structures for nonspeech movements should be assessed by speech-language professionals. For those leery of the use of the term *oral apraxia,* we suggest that *descriptions* of behaviors demonstrated during nonspeech tasks can be extremely helpful in documenting problems, or lack of same, with the functional adequacy of these structures. This may provide a helpful alternative to diagnostic labeling of the disorder.

The *Volitional Oral Movements* examination, originally published by Darley and Spriestersbach (1978), has been a helpful tool for us in evaluating non-speech function of the speech mechanism. The instrument incorporates both isolated and sequenced movements as well as a scale which rates how independently the client is able to perform the tasks. It should be noted that Prichard, Tekieli, and Kozup (1979) found that both isolated and sequenced volitional oral movement tasks differentiated their three developmentally apraxic subjects from age-matched controls with functional articulation disorders.

It has been our experience that diadochokinetic tasks can be particularly helpful in evaluating the stability of repeated nonspeech movements. These tasks should be specifically designed to stress the use of the mechanism for nonspeech movements by complexity of the requested movements and by multiple trials. The children we evaluate typically demonstrate deterioration in accuracy and smoothness of the movements during successive diadochokinetic trials. Thus a child who can adequately perform an initial trial of the "tongue wiggle" (alternately touching the corners of the mouth with the tongue tip) may experience many more problems with the task when attempting it on the second or third trial. We also find a child's ability to perform the "tongue circle" (following the lips in a circular movement) helpful in assessing a child's ability to control tongue movements. Frequently, the children with DAS seem to have tongues that are "lost" in their mouths, unable to smoothly follow the lips in a circular movement, which, of course, necessitates a constant change in the direction of the tongue movements. An additional observation we have made during examinations of nonspeech oral movement adequacy is that children with DAS occasionally will use their fingers to manipulate their lips and tongues in their attempts to monitor or complete the requested movement(s).

Instrumental tests of articulator movement may also be useful in evaluating the child with DAS. Such tasks as fine force control (McNeil, Weismer, Adams, & Mulligan, 1990) or visuomotor tracking (McClean, Buekelman, & Yorkston, 1987; Moon, Robin, Zebrowski, & Folkins, 1991) have been used to study the coordination of the articulators with apraxic or dysarthric speakers as well as with children who stutter. Such tasks may be useful in documenting the presence and extent of oral apraxia in children with speech sound problems.

Auditory Processing Problems

Throughout the history of DAS, numerous authors have addressed the auditory processing abilities of these children (e.g., Eisenson, 1972; Morley, 1959; Orton, 1937). However, data on auditory perceptual skills in children with DAS are scarce. Table 6.5 summarizes the findings from the data-based studies with children exhibiting DAS in which some level of auditory perception was examined. One consistent finding is that the auditory acuity for pure tone stimuli is normal. This is not surprising since normal hearing is often used as an inclusion criterion in studies involving children with DAS. Other aspects of auditory perception that have been tested include auditory discrimination, sound recognition, auditory memory, and auditory sequencing abilities. As is apparent from Table 6.5, a range of severity levels has been reported.

Assessment

While certainly auditory problems can occur in DAS and auditory status should be included in the overall picture of an individual child, these dis-

TABLE 6.5
Auditory Processing Skills of Children with DAS

DATA-BASED STUDY	CHILDREN WITH DAS	AUDITORY TESTS	RESULTS
Eisenson, 1972	1	response to environmental sounds	normal
Yoss & Darley, 1974a	30	*Denver Auditory Phonemic Sequencing Test*	Significantly poorer than normal
Prichard, Tekieli, & Kozup, 1979	6	*Goldman-Fristoe-Woodcock Auditory Skills Test*	below normal for: Selective Attention Diagnostic Discrimination Recognition Memory Memory for Sequence Sound Recognition
Williams & Ingham, 1981	30	*Denver Auditory Phonemic Sequencing Test*	normal (although authors note that 3 children with DAS greater than 1 SD from mean of normal
Love & Fitzgerald, 1984	1	*Goldman-Fristoe-Woodcock Auditory Skills Test*	below normal for: Selective Attention Sound Discrimination Sound Blending
Robin, Hall, & Jordan, 1986	5	Robin 6-Element Temporal Processing Task	below normal

orders are considered to be concomitant with the apraxia. In general, the data suggest that, while hearing thresholds for pure tones are within normal limits, children with DAS often have difficulty with more complex auditory perceptual tasks such as environmental sound discrimination and speech discrimination. Tests that have been used to assess auditory functioning in children exhibiting DAS include the *Denver Auditory Phonemic Sequencing Test,* (Aten, 1979) and the *Goldman-Fristoe-Woodcock Auditory Skills Battery* (Goldman, Fristoe, & Woodcock, 1974). Robin (Robin, Hall, & Jordan, 1986; Robin, Tomblin, Kearney, & Hug, 1989; Robin, Tranel, & Damasio, 1990) has developed a test that specifically examines auditory temporal processing in six element patterns. Such tests may provide the clinician with information pertaining to the auditory processing skills of a given child with DAS.

Psychological Factors: Intelligence

Several authors have discussed the intellectual abilities of children with DAS. McGinnis (1963) listed intelligence within the normal range as a characteristic of children with *motor aphasia.* Later in the text, McGinnis more completely described the children as ranging in intelligence from "dull normal to slightly above normal levels. There were few with superior intelligence" (p. 35). Marquardt and Sussman (1991) stated "decreased intellectual functioning does not appear to be a characteristic distinctive to DAS" (p. 348).

Two empirical studies used intellectual abilities as a subject selection criterion and illustrate the wide range of possible intelligence defined as average or above. Yoss and Darley (1974b) established a subject criterion of an intelligence quotient of 90 or above for inclusion in their study. The 30 "defective articulation children" (those with DAS) were reported to have tested intelligence quotients ranging from 90 to 122, with a median score of 103. Aram and Horwitz (1981) used a criterion of normal nonverbal intelligence, defined as a score of 80 or above, for subject inclusion. They reported a range of scores from 83 to 130 in their 10 subjects. In contrast, the Ferry, Hall, and Hicks (1975) clinical report on *developmental verbal dyspraxia* did not use a predetermined intellectual criterion in their subject selection process. Their findings included a range of intelligence levels, which encompassed individuals functioning with I.Q.s between 40 and 120 in 60 subjects.

Previously mentioned studies on genetic factors relating to DAS (see Chapter 5) also included information about intellectual status. These studies will now be discussed in more detail. The Ferry et al. study provides additional information that needs to be noted: Two of the 60 subjects with *developmental verbal dyspraxia* were reported to have Down Syndrome, a syndrome in which mental retardation is typically exhibited.

McLaughlin and Kriegsmann (1980) reported the occurrence of developmental dyspraxia in two subjects exhibiting Renpenning Syndrome. One of the subjects described in the report obtained a full scale IQ of 45 on the *Wechsler Intelligence Scale for Children–Revised* (WISC–R) (Wechsler, 1974), with no split between the verbal and performance scores. The second subject, a half- brother of the first subject, achieved an IQ equivalent of 60 on the *McCarthy Perceptual-Performance Scale of Children's Abilities* (McCarthy, 1972) and an IQ of 97 on the *Arthur Adaptation of the Leiter International Performance Scale* (Arthur, 1952). Paul, Cohen, Breg, Watson, and Herman (1984) described three patients with fragile X Syndrome who also exhibited DAS. The nonverbal intelligence quotients of the patients were 40, 50, and 70 as determined by the *Leiter International Performance Scale* (Arthur, 1952), and the WISC–R (Wechsler, 1974). These three studies point out the reported occurrence of DAS in special populations of children, including those who function within the mentally retarded range of intellectual potential.

A child's intellectual test scores are generally considered to be a measure of achievement and a predictor of future potential. The psychologist who tests the child exhibiting DAS must be trained with a variety of instruments so that a verbal instrument is not used until the child has some degree of intelligibility. Nevertheless, the limitations of a performance only measure must be recognized. The psychologist may need to rely on the speech-language pathologist for help in the testing of the child with poor intelligibility or with the child who relies heavily on signs or gestures. Intelligence test score profiles may be helpful in designing or selecting a remedial program. Observations made during testing, when teamed with those of the speech-language pathologist made during initial remediation sessions, are helpful in attempting to describe a child's learning style. Measurement of levels of intellectual functioning are also helpful in arriving at estimates of prognosis of the eventual communication status that a child with DAS will achieve. Communication skills do not develop or exist in a vacuum. Estimates of intelligence are also useful in predicting the eventual skills and abilities the individual is capable of developing for dealing with the world as he or she strives for independence.

We have followed children with DAS who present a wide range of intellectual abilities. The child's formal intellectual test results often reflect large gaps or splits between their verbal and performance abilities, with the performance skills usually being the stronger ones. A psychologist skilled in dealing with children with severe communication disorders is an invaluable member of the team working with a child presenting DAS. Reliable performance intelligence scores may be obtained with the young or severely disordered child. Later, increased intelligibility will allow the psychologist to reliably transcribe verbal responses in order to gain an estimate of verbal intelligence.

Psychological Factors: Personality and Behavior

Orton (1937) was the first to address the personalities of children he had studied who exhibited "motor speech delays." He described the children as having a "quiet, friendly shyness", and noted they responded to social contacts although they did not initiate such contacts due to their difficulty in expressing themselves. Orton further noted that the children did not seem to have abnormal fears and were not seclusive, although they often demonstrated marked reactions to frustration due to difficulties in making themselves understood. Morley (1957) reported little evidence of emotional disturbances in her discussion of children with developmental articulatory apraxia. However, she noted increased reticence and hesitation to talk as the children became more aware of their problems in making themselves understood. She further noted that as speech improvement occurred, the children seemed to experience a decrease in anxiety about talking as well as increases in self-confidence. Morley concluded that she did not think psychogenic factors played a part in this particular speech disorder.

On a less positive note, Ferry, Hall, and Hicks (1975) reported that almost all of the 60 *verbally dyspraxic* children included in their study, 20 of whom were residents of a state institution for mentally retarded individuals, had significant behavioral or emotional problems; 32 had temper tantrums, 14 suffered depression, and four were autistic. However, we suggest that the cited behavioral and emotional problems may not be related solely to the children's reported dyspraxia. Rapin and Allen (1981) described children with *phonologic programming deficit syndrome* and also noted that a variety of behavioral disorders may be exhibited, resulting from the frustration of ineffective communication abilities. While Blakeley (1983) does not consider DAS to be a behavioral anomaly, he noted behaviors such as temper tantrums, inflexibility, distractibility, aggression, excessive motor activity and withdrawal, which he thought were due to difficulties in being understood.

We believe that DAS occurs in children, not in a special type of child. As a result, DAS occurs in children who exhibit a variety of personality profiles, emotional states, and behavioral patterns. By far the majority of the children we have seen appear to be *normal* children in many ways. They are frequently very diligent and persistent in their willingness to work with speech-language pathologists to improve their communication skills. Rosenbek (1985) observed that adult "apraxic patients are notoriously hard working. Even small gains in functional communication are enough to make them increase their efforts" (p. 298). We often find the same to be true of children with DAS. However, even the most tolerant children seem to have limits in the amount of frustration with which they can deal. Thus, clinicians working with children exhibiting DAS must be sensitive about, and have the counseling skills necessary, to appropriately respond to the children's overt and covert expressions of frustration and occasional anger.

CHAPTER 7

Remediation: Motor-Programming Approaches to DAS

Methodological Problems

In previous chapters we have discussed the speech characteristics that are frequently used to describe DAS as well as methods used to assess these characteristics. Also presented were theories that might explain the underlying problems related to control of the oral mechanism during the speech efforts of children experiencing DAS. Further, we have described a number of behaviors that often co-occur in children who exhibit DAS. Once a clinician has considered a diagnosis of developmental apraxia of speech, the challenge becomes one of how to best treat the disorder. This challenge is complex.

Previously we mentioned the common observation that children with DAS respond very slowly to intervention procedures. Clinicians report that they have been required to put a great deal of time, thought, and effort into their programming for these children. When something seemed to "work" many of these practitioners have graciously shared this information with others in the profession. Thus, a number of philosophies, remedial ideas, and specific techniques exist in the body of literature dealing with DAS. However, as with other aspects of this complex disorder, there does not appear to be universal acceptance of the potential answers to treatment questions.

A number of factors must be taken into consideration when critically analyzing treatment literature. The number of children for whom any particular treatment has been successful is often quite limited, if reported at all. Much of the treatment literature consists of case studies involving only one or two subjects. To further complicate this issue, many of these are retrospective studies, and actual data regarding ongoing trends in the acquisition of speech skills are lost. Moreover, most reports of treatment contained in case studies did not use research designs that allow for evaluation of the efficacy of a given treatment approach. Such may not be the case when research methodologies consistent with single-subject designs are used. Many times other intervention techniques are briefly described, without specific information being provided as to how many children with DAS (or other communication disorders) had been treated and had experienced success with the technique or program. The literature to date presents information that has not typically been studied systematically or studied on a small number of children who present the disorder. Thus generalization of a given treatment approach to other children with DAS has not been possible.

Characteristics of the subject(s) to consider when evaluating the present intervention literature include age, the severity of the DAS, and potential effects of previous and accompanying treatment approaches. Complicating the picture with DAS in relation to the issue of age, of course, is the fact that many of the children are seen in the age range when communication skills are still developing. In addition, the success of any treatment approach may be related to the severity of the subjects' communication disorder and their responsiveness to remedial techniques. A child with a more mild degree of DAS involvement may (or may not) respond more quickly and positively to a technique than a child with a severe DAS involvement. The child's experiences with prior remediation may influence a technique under study. Previously acquired skills or knowledge, attitudes, and motivation to succeed may have been shaped by earlier treatment experiences. These are all major factors to consider when developing any remedial program. Consideration must be given to comparability between the research population being reviewed and any particular client for whom a remedial approach is being selected.

Some of the techniques reported in the literature lack sufficient description to allow another person to use them and thus to replicate the initial research efforts. The success of such techniques may be solely dependant on the skill of the clinician who develops them and may fall into the "art" of the profession. Some techniques have prospered as long as the clinician developing them is able to directly teach others how to use them, becoming a mentor for others. However, none, to our knowledge, have been exposed to the rigors of efficacy studies.

It is our premise that the DAS treatment literature frequently lacks objectivity in the measurement of the behaviors targeted for modification. Conclusions regarding the effectiveness of remediation are often based on the clinician's subjective observations and impressions; the conclusions have seldom been reached by the systematic gathering of experimental evidence. The study of remediation of children with DAS is in its infancy, and hopefully as more knowledge is gained about the disorder, the treatment needs will be identified and efficacy of treatment will be demonstrated.

The remainder of this chapter and Chapter 8 will present information regarding a number (we did not attempt to be exhaustive) of remedial/

treatment/therapy/intervention (we use the terms interchangeably) techniques that are currently available and have been reported to be helpful to speech-language professionals in their work with the *speech* aspects of the communication problems presented by children with DAS.

Motor-Programming Approaches to DAS Remediation

As we have written at numerous junctures in earlier parts of this text, we view DAS as a disorder of motor control during speech production. When asked specifically to do so, the child may be unable to replicate the movements of the speech producing mechanism, even though he or she may well be able to spontaneously or unconsciously make these movements. Because we view the problem as one of motor control, our remedial philosophy, after identifying a child in whom we think DAS may be the presenting problem, is that of designing motor-program based intervention for the child (Hall, 1992). Inherent in this philosophy is the remedial goal for the child with DAS to acquire *voluntary, accurate,* and *consistent* control of the speech articulators so that phonemes and phoneme sequences are produced accurately and consistently when the child voluntarily decides, or is asked, to do so.

There is no single source or reference to which readers can be referred that covers all the various components and tenants that individual authors consider to constitute motor-programming therapy. Many of the remediation concepts that are called motor-programming originated in the literature dealing with the rehabilitation of adult apraxics. The etiology for the apraxia in the adult population is documentable, in sharp contrast with children exhibiting the developmental form of the disorder. However, many of the theories, principles, and hierarchies described for work with adult apraxics are potentially helpful to the clinician designing a motor-programming remedial program for an *individual* child. (We stress the word "individual" since the program development for children with DAS must meet the individual, and often unique, needs of each child.) Authors who have written about remediation with adult apraxic patients include Darley, Aronson, and Brown (1975); Dabul and Bollier (1976); Rosenbek (1985); Hagen (1987); and Rosenbek, Kent, and LaPointe (1984).

Within the literature dealing with DAS and remediation, Hadden (1891) can be credited with publication of the initial thoughts on intervention. In his case study he wrote descriptions of the instructional techniques used with Charles M., which included many of the concepts that would be included in a motor-programming approach today. Morley (1957, 1965, 1972) also addressed the treatment approach and needs of the apraxic child, with many suggestions being consistent with motor-programming. The publications of Chappell (1973); Yoss and Darley (1974b); and Rosenbek, Hansen, Baughman, and Lemme (1974) heralded an increase in the number of contributions in the literature about the disorder itself, as well as suggested ways with which the disorder could be treated. This included use of motor-programming approaches.

Features of Motor-Programming Approaches

The articles written on motor-programming therapy with DAS present collections of principles and modes of operation. The resultant program developed by a clinician for a particular client is probably an eclectic collection of what seems to best fit that particular child. However, to our knowledge, the efficacy of treatment programs with children exhibiting DAS that purport to be motor-program-based has not yet been tested. The most salient features of what we refer to as motor-programming approaches to therapy with a child exhibiting DAS are the following:

1. Intensive services are needed.

2. Many repetitions of speech movements are needed, elicited in drill-oriented sessions.

3. Remediation should progress systematically through hierarchies of task difficulty.

4. Remediation should stress sequences of movements, and the development of the "memory" for such movement patterns.

5. The clinician should determine the need for auditory discrimination tasks in the remedial program.

6. Remediation should include emphasis on self-monitoring.

7. The clinician should use input from multiple modalities.

8. Remediation should include manipulation of prosodic features as an integral part of the total remedial program.

9. The clinician should, if necessary, teach compensatory strategies.

10. The clinician must provide successful experiences.

We will now explore each of these features more completely.

INTENSIVE SERVICES ARE NEEDED FOR THE CHILD WITH DAS.   Children with DAS are reported to make slow progress in the remediation of their speech problem. They seem to require a great deal of professional service, typically done on an individual basis. Therefore, clinicians working with DAS must accommodate this need and schedule as much intervention time with the child as the child and/or his/her circumstances can allow. Thus, the clinician may be thrust into the position of becoming an advocate on behalf of the child to assure that services are provided as frequently as possible. In some cases, the clinician may need to help the family find the financial resources or assistance they may need to cover the costs of professional service; a child with DAS can quickly become an expensive child to his/her family or school system because of the amount of therapy they typically require.

The roles of parents, teachers, peers, and siblings in a child's program of remediation will also vary with the circumstances. If the child with DAS can tolerate additional work and interacts well with the selected individual, the speech-language pathologist may include family and/or teachers in the overall programming to provide additional response opportunities for the child to reinforce and strengthen performance on a particular speech target. Creaghead, Newman, and Secord (1989) stated that "nightly parental drill . . . is a necessity" (p. 274). However, in today's society we recognize that the involvement of the family and teachers in the extra remedial programming may not be a practical recommendation to pursue.

The definition of "intensive" varies from clinician to clinician and from work setting to work setting. Rosenbek (1985), when discussing therapy with adult apraxics, defines the word as meaning that the patient and the clinician should have daily sessions; Macaluso-Haynes (1978), Haynes (1985), and Blakeley (1983) also advocate daily remediation sessions. Blakeley (1983, p. 27) stated that "I do not expect to provide speech education for children with developmental apraxia of speech on a cursory basis for it may be the most important part of their entire education." Our use of the word reflects a programming option available in our clinic, which includes a summer program where children are in residence for 6 weeks, receiving 4 hours of remediation for 5 days each week. It is our experience that these intensive summer sessions result in greater gains in remedial goals than children with DAS experience when they receive services once or twice weekly for half-hour or hourly sessions.

MANY REPETITIONS OF SPEECH MOVEMENTS ARE NEEDED, ELICITED IN DRILL-ORIENTED SESSIONS.   The purpose of the numerous repetitions of particular speech movements is to increase the child's volitional control over the movement patterns. This is important so that "ingraining and habituation of accurate motor planning for speech" (Macaluso-Haynes, 1978, p. 247) can take place. Numerous repetitions are also consistent with theories of motor learning (Schmidt, 1988). This therapy feature is accomplished by developing remedial sessions that are highly response-oriented, with numerous response opportunities being afforded the child. There need to be a number of repetitions of speech movements, whether the repetition is of a CV syllable or a multisyllabic word. We tend to incorporate 3 to 10 repetitions of the stimuli into our therapy activities, although some clinicians with whom we have exchanged ideas report that they have demanded as many as 20 repetitions. Perhaps the actual number of repetitions needs to be determined with the child's proficiency level and tolerance for the task being prime considerations. It is thought that these repetitions place desirable stress upon the speech motor system and assist in the development and maintenance of accurate speech movement sequences.

Another premise that we use in our clinical work is to assure that the client comes to a resting or neutral position between each repetition of a response set. We have observed that some children, once they have obtained correct placement of the articulators, may set them into that position in an attempt to duplicate their success. In order for the child to maximally benefit from the remediation, we require them to come to a resting position after a response before the next one is attempted.

We think that perceptual accuracy is essential and needs to be the criterion by which responses are judged correct or incorrect by the clinician. Recall that the child with DAS has a capacity to produce extremely subtle errors. Almost getting the correct voicing on an attempted /b/ should not be reinforced as a correct /b/. We do not want the child programmed to habitually use the almost-but-not-quite-correct production. The only exception to demand of accuracy in production trials might involve the shaping of selected phonemes. For example, with several children we have seen, we decided that it was important for a child to have an /s/-marker in their morphology for language work, even though it was a distorted /s/. A later goal worked to shape the /s/ toward the non-distorted standard production of the phoneme.

Macaluso-Haynes (1978) makes a good suggestion about dealing with possible perseverative behavior during the intensive and repetitive speech work necessitated by a motor-programming approach to remediation. She suggests that potential perseveration can be reduced if the drill is interrupted periodically for a rest period or by changing the activities which are being used. Rosenbek, Hansen, Baughman, and Lemme (1974) suggest that the drills used in remediation be blocked rather than massed. Thus they suggest limiting the amount of time spent on drill activities or the number of repetitions of individual stimuli.

REMEDIATION SHOULD PROGRESS SYSTEMATICALLY THROUGH HIERAR-CHIES OF TASK DIFFICULTY. The learning principle of beginning with the most simple task and slowly building task difficulty until the most complex task is accomplished is very apropos for work with children exhibiting DAS.

We are in agreement with Morley (1957) who stated that "treatment will depend on what the child can do" (p. 265). There are a variety of suggestions as well as points of disagreement in the literature on the issue of where to begin with a client exhibiting DAS. Considerations presented in the literature to help determine the task level at which to initially establish goals include the following:

SHOULD USE OF TONGUE AND LIP STRENGTHENING AND MOVEMENT EXERCISES SERVE AS PRECURSORS TO DIRECT WORK ON SPEECH PRODUCTION? Macaluso-Haynes (1978) and Haynes (1985) suggested providing concentrated drill on tongue and lip movements, both in imitated activities and to command. She further suggested that these be done in both isolation and in sequences. Yoss and Darley (1974b) also advocated use of these types of activities in an effort to reduce the degree of oral apraxia that may be present. They suggest initial mirror work with reinforcement provided for movements that demonstrate good range and placement accuracy and are performed immediately and accurately upon request with no searching or extraneous movements. There are no data to suggest that strengthening exercises are efficacious as part of a treatment program for children with developmental apraxia. Even the data on strength training for subjects with dysarthria are controversial at best.

It should be pointed out that the relationship between speech and nonspeech movements of the articulators has not been adequately addressed in the literature. While Robin (1992) argued that apraxic children should benefit from training of nonspeech movement patterns of the articulators, no data to date address this issue. The extant literature has shown a relationship between speech and nonspeech movements, depending on the nonspeech task employed. For example, Hixon and Hardy (1964) did not find a correlation between nonspeech oral movements and speech in individuals diagnosed with cerebral palsy. However, Barlow and Abbs (1986) found a strong correlation between fine force and position control tasks and speech intelligibility scores in subjects diagnosed with upper motor neuron syndrome. Since the ability to imitate any movement may be problematic for some children with apraxia, it may be desirable to include these types of activities in early stages of remediation, but with the rationale that the objective is to help the child learn to imitate movement patterns and not to improve the oral apraxia that may also be present.

Related to the issue of treatment of nonspeech movement patterns is the question as to whether or not oral apraxia should be targeted as a treatment goal. Remediation of oral apraxia is not necessarily a goal we would endorse, depending on a given child and his/her needs. Since oral apraxia does co-occur with apraxia of speech, some clinicians may feel the need to remediate this aspect of the child's disorder. However, remediation of oral apraxia in and of itself may not facilitate the acquisition of motor programming for speech production purposes. While the treatment of movement patterns discussed above may affect both the oral and speech apraxias, remediation of the oral apraxia without reference to speech motor control may not facilitate speech improvement. Thus, we reiterate that treatment of movement patterns should be specifically aimed at the acquisition of speech movements. As such, nonspeech movement patterns that relate to speech control need to be developed and then their applicability to speech remediation should be tested.

SHOULD WORK BEGIN WITH PHONEMES IN ISOLATION? Marquardt and Sussman (1991) suggested that with severely disordered children with DAS it may be necessary to begin intervention at the individual phoneme level so that motor control is achieved on the speech sounds in isolation. In fact, the more typical beginning level of work is with the nonsense syllable such as CV combinations because of the necessity of producing consonants with a releasing vowel. On the other hand, there are also those who suggest that work on production of phonemes in isolation should be avoided: Rosenbek, Hansen, Baughman, and Lemme (1974) describe the isolated sound as "elusive," while Weiss, Gordon, and Lillywhite (1987) suggest that production training should emphasize sequences, so work should begin with CV and VC syllables, rather than phonemes in isolation.

WHICH PHONEMES SHOULD BE SELECTED FOR INITIAL REMEDIATION EFFORTS?
Vowels. Chappell (1973) recommended that the vowels /o/, /a/, /i/, and /æ/ be included in the initial group of targeted phonemes. Yoss and Darley (1974b) suggested that following the previously discussed tongue and lip exercises, the initial speech goal would be imitated sustained vowels with exaggerated lip movement and mandibular range of movement. Blakeley, in his 1983 DAS treatment program based on the need to improve overall intelligibility, included the teaching of vowels early in the intervention process. This was based on the observation that vowel errors significantly interfere with listener intelligibility. While we readily acknowledge the validity of this premise, we have not had good success with the remediation of this group of phonemes, regardless of where in the sequence of remediation they are targeted. Vowel remediation seems to be relatively unaddressed in our field. We do not typically target vowels, specifically, in the early phases of our intervention programs with children presenting DAS, although we do use and reinforce vowels that occur spontaneously in the child's vocal productions.
Early developing consonants. Blakeley (1983) suggested that the early developed consonants should be targeted initially. This was based on the impression that the motor patterns necessary for earlier developing con-

sonants were easier than in later learned sounds, and that the consonants were used in the production of early learned words.

Frequently occurring consonants. With the goal of improved intelligibility, Blakeley (1983) suggested targeting those consonants that are frequently occurring within the language. He thought that the incorporation of these phonemes would increase intelligibility to greater extents than would the targeting of sounds that occur less frequently. Such a strategy also increases the corpus of words with which to work in remediation, and thus the child with DAS has more frequent opportunities to produce the targeted phonemes.

Visible consonants. Yoss and Darley (1974b) suggested the initial step in consonant work be that of imitating the visible consonants, which should then to be paired with the vowels already in the child's repertoire for CV and VC level work. Rosenbek, Hansen, Baughman, and Lemme (1974) also advocated targeting visible consonants first, such as /p/, /t/, and /f/, followed by the nasals and then the /b/, /d/, and /v/. Macaluso-Haynes (1978) noted that selection of visible phonemes "may give rapid initial success" (p. 246). Blakeley (1983) suggested introduction of visibly produced sounds because he thought that the visual modality of children with DAS was facilitative in the remedial process. He listed the most visible phonemes as /m/, /p/, /b/, /f/, /v/, /θ/, /ð/, /n/, /t/, /d/, /l/, /tʃ/, /dʒ/, /s/, and /z/. Consideration of a phoneme's visibility during production was also advocated by Marquardt, Dunn, and Davis (1985); Weiss, Gordon, and Lillywhite (1987); and Marquardt and Sussman (1991).

VOICELESS CONSONANTS. Chappell (1973); Rosenbek, Hansen, Baughman, and Lemme (1974); Macaluso-Haynes (1978); Weiss, Gordon, and Lillywhite (1987); and Marquardt and Sussman (1991) all suggested that voiceless consonants should be presented to the child with apraxia before voiced phonemes are targeted. In our remedial work we find that we agree with Blakeley's (1983) more temperate position that "voiceless sounds may be easier to teach" (p. 29). It was his position that voiced phonemes require greater motor speech skills than do voiceless phonemes, and he advocated that each child be assessed so that "each is taught according to his or her most rapid learning skills" (p. 29). Although the voiceless phonemes may be easier to produce, pairing such voiceless phonemes with vowels (which requires use of voice) presents an error-fraught situation that may tax the speech motor control of a child with DAS.

Although many suggestions have been offered by many clinicians on how to establish initial remedial goals, there appears to be no one set of guidelines accepted by all practitioners for all children with DAS. We are most confident in the path determined by careful observation and assessment of each child's strengths.

Progression of remediation using motor-programming approaches follows an expanded version of those steps included in traditional articulation intervention. However, the steps within the traditional therapy model must be *extremely* carefully manipulated into small steps to accommodate the production competencies of the individual child with DAS. A student clinician of ours once stated he felt he was breaking the remedial steps into "subatomic" levels to adequately meet the needs of his client. The increases in the complexity of responses demanded from the child progress slowly, but in a controlled fashion. Typically, remediation with a child presenting DAS consists initially of many repetitions of single movements, followed by simple movement sequences and later by more complicated movement sequences. Examples of this type of careful progression of remedial steps are provided by Morley and Fox (1969) and Morley (1972).

An example of the meticulousness with which a clinician may need to plan the early levels of an intervention program will now be presented using a client (W.J.) as an example.

- Using information obtained during an initial assessment regarding W. J.'s articulatory skills, it was observed that he could produce the /m/, /d/, /a/, and /ʌ/ phonemes with some degree of success. These were targeted for production in isolation until he was consistent in his ability to produce them volitionally and upon command (non-imitated and non-modeled responses).

- Subsequently these phonemes were combined into CV, then VC sequences, each new combination occurring after consistency had been achieved with the previous type of phoneme combination. Reduplicated syllables (CVCV, VCVC) were included in this sequence to expand the number of phonemes included in the syllable shape. The sequences were then alternated (CV VC, CV VC).

- Next W. J. was asked to produce CVC and C_1VC_2-type sequences. Although Edwards (1973) suggested that "too early use of words may serve to reinforce former deviant patterns" (p. 69), we try to include as many real words as could be developed from the targeted phonemes, since the use of real words would give W. J., and his parents a sense that he really can produce meaningful words correctly. This also gives any client some degree of power and verbal control over his world. The use of real words early in the remedial process is a position shared by Chappell (1973), who suggested that soon after the initiation of therapy "a few monosyllabic words of high utility" (p. 366) be incorporated into the program. Yoss and Darley (1974b) suggested use of real and nonsense rhyming words as minimal pairs when this level of remediation is reached. Lohr (1978) suggested using words that are important and useful to the child, while Blakeley (1983) suggested using frequently occurring words that will aid in over-all improvement of intelligibility. His suggestions were that words from the child's environment, and therefore presumably important to the child, should be targeted. Blakeley also suggested that word lists, such as from reading programs, could also be of assistance in developing speech stimulus lists. Perhaps frequency of occurrence of words that are used in the child's environment could also be helpful in determining words of high potential communication value.

- W. J.'s remedial program was next expanded by including more phonemes in the syllable and word shapes, these phonemes having been elicited and stabilized at the isolation level while work on the /m/, /d/, /a/, and /ʌ/ phonemes was in the earlier stages of syllable work. The syllables included combinations of several different consonants and vowels and were expanded to include $C_1V_1C_2V_2C_1$ and similar syllable/word constructions.

- This process continued, with expansion into higher levels of complexity using multisyllabic words of 2-5 syllables in length and words that contained consonant clusters in various word positions.

- These words could then be placed into carrier phrases, patterned sentences, imitated and original sentences, etc. These levels of remediation also need to be carefully controlled for task complexity as to length of the total utterance and placement of targeted words within them. Finally, whole utterance accuracy needs to be targeted and achieved.

Several factors that we consider important are illustrated by W. J.'s therapy program. We included prosodic goals, which will be discussed in more detail later in the chapter, at each level of articulatory work. As discussed in Chapter 2, children with DAS may be dysprosodic and we think that recognition and modification of this facet of communication is necessary, and should be dealt with in tandem with speech goals. A second factor to recall is that, by it's very nature, apraxia is a speech disorder that is inconsistent. Clinicians working with children demonstrating DAS must be alert to highly variable and inconsistent performances within sessions and from one intervention session to the next. Therefore, it is incumbent upon clinicians to remain flexible in their goal setting for any individual session—plans need to be modified according to the level at which the client can succeed during any particular moment on any particular day. A third factor involved in this model of remediation is that it needs to maintain sensitivity to goals that involve disordered language such as attention to syntax at the sentence level. A final point we need to stress is that remedial programs will probably proceed extremely slowly, even with intensive services. Children with DAS need to produce *many* response repetitions at each level and often with every minute change in the difficulty level of the targeted responses. The definition of *many* response repetitions will need to be determined with each client exhibiting DAS.

Clinicians may also need to give some thought to the number of stimuli used at each level of remediation. Rosenbek, Hansen, Baughman, and Lemme (1974) and Weiss, Gordon, and Lillywhite (1987) suggest that a limited number of stimuli should be used with children exhibiting DAS. Weiss et al. state that the use of "too many stimuli can be confusing . . . by providing competing stimuli [they] cancel or reduce the effects of the preferred sensory modality" (p. 264). We do not think that this restriction necessarily applies to remediation with every child with DAS. While an individual child may initially benefit from a small "core" of stimuli, we are hopeful that this restriction is necessary only when a new level of difficulty is introduced to the child. Our impression is that as speech proficiency improves, the stimulus pool should be expanded so that the child has the opportunity to gain articulator control over a larger number of phonemes and phoneme sequences.

REMEDIATION SHOULD STRESS SEQUENCES OF MOVEMENTS, AND THE DEVELOPMENT OF THE "MEMORY" FOR SUCH MOVEMENT PATTERNS. The outline of remediation just presented describes the need for the careful incremental increase in the difficulty level of the stimuli and expected response, which is done for the purpose of carefully sequencing the difficulty in the movements of speech. Rosenbek, Hansen, Baughman, and Lemme (1974) state that "as a general principle, therapy, from the beginning, should emphasize movement sequences regardless of the severity of the apraxia" (p. 14). Chappell (1973) stated "memory for articulation behavior . . . consists of an internalized and assimilated system based on tactile-kinesthetic-proprioceptive information which explicitly relates heard sound with speech-motor patterns" (p. 364). He provided suggestions for the development, establishment, and retention of memory for articulation patterns. This includes the use of "chaining" and "backward chaining" for developing and establishing movement sequences. He also suggested increasing the demand for memory retention by providing interruptions between requests for responses and opportunities for their actual production. Weiss, Gordon, and Lillywhite (1987) state that the memory for articulatory movements must be demonstrated in volitional and not imitative movements.

THE CLINICIAN SHOULD DETERMINE THE NEED FOR AUDITORY DISCRIMINATION TASKS IN THE REMEDIAL PROGRAM. Our experience with children exhibiting DAS is that they are usually abundantly aware of the phonemes that they are unable to articulate or that they misarticulate. Their auditory discrimination skills are often well developed, which may contribute to their frustration. Unless a child has clearly demonstrated that they are not able to identify the presence of a phoneme or to make discriminations between several with similar acoustic properties, we do not use valuable remediation time for these types of activities. This philosophy is shared by Yoss and Darley (1974b); Macaluso-Haynes (1978) Haynes (1985); and Weiss, Gordon, and Lillywhite (1987). On the other hand, Chappell (1973) writes that in his experience with children demonstrating DAS there is failure with auditory discrimination skills, thus he encourages the inclusion of this feature in remedial planning. As with many aspects of DAS, there are differences of opinion about problems in auditory discrimination skills and what to do about this in the clinical setting.

REMEDIATION SHOULD EMPHASIZE SELF-MONITORING. Perhaps the most important skill for any client with a speech sound disorder is the ability to monitor themselves in order to identify correct productions and to modify errored ones. This skill also extends to the child with DAS. We think that auditory self-monitoring is a very important aspect of remediation, even for those children who seem to otherwise have good auditory discrimination. "Many children have good ability to discriminate interpersonally, but on an intrapersonal basis they fail lamentably" (Edwards, 1973, p. 69). We too observe that some of our DAS clients find it easier to identify speech errors made by other speakers than those they themselves make.

While we most frequently use auditory self-evaluation tasks to help achieve the self-monitoring goal in remediation, other types of self-monitoring come into play more subtly. Weiss, Gordan, and Lillywhite (1987) suggest that tactile and kinesthetic self-monitoring be trained. Other authors are less specific as to the types of self-monitoring that should be included within the therapy program (Macaluso-Haynes, 1978; Marquardt, Dunn, & Davis, 1985; Air, Wood, & Neils, 1989).

Yoss and Darley (1974b) suggest that self-monitoring of spontaneous speech should be introduced as early as possible within the remedial framework, noting that slowing rate may be necessary in order to achieve this goal. We agree that self-monitoring of spontaneous speech is the ultimate goal and that the skills need to be developed from the earliest, simplest level of speech production. This must be emphasized until the individual child is capable of self-monitoring his/her own spontaneous speech.

THE CLINICIAN SHOULD USE INPUT FROM MULTIPLE MODALITIES. Children with DAS often seem to require a great deal of assistance in helping them produce and sequence phonemes. Often times the assistance that seems most helpful are cues utilizing various senses. Thus, in addition to our often used auditory cues, the clients with DAS may find cues presented in visual, tactile, and kinesthetic modalities (frequently used in combination) helpful because these increase orosensory and/or auditory perceptual awareness. Our philosophy is to use what works to achieve the goals, although the clinician must work with each individual child to determine what type(s) of cueing is most facilitating for him/her.

The use of multisensory input has been suggested by numerous authors, starting with Hadden in 1891. Morley (1957, 1965, 1972); Eisenson (1972); Blakeley (1983); Yoss and Darley (1974b); Lohr (1978); Rosenbek, Hansen, Baughman, and Lemme (1974); Weiss, Gordon, and Lillywhite (1987); and Marquardt & Sussman (1991) suggest use of the visual modality in such activities as imitation, where the child watches the clinician's oral movements and attempts to replicate the movement. Tactile cueing was suggested by Morley and Fox (1969); Eisenson (1972); Lohr (1978); Blakeley (1983); Marquardt, Dunn, and Davis (1985); and Marquardt and Sussman (1991). The various types of cuing discussed in this literature involve such things as use of spatulas, tongue depressors, probe sticks, teaspoons, application of various textures, swabbing, and pressure touches to help the child by actual manipulation of the tongue to assist in the needed lingual movements or to provide cues of articulator placement or movement direction. Tactile cuing can also be helpful in achieving the correct voicing feature. For instance, we have used an electrolarynx to help a child learn the contrast between voicing and voicelessness in cognate phoneme pairs (Jordan, 1988).

There are a number of specific remedial techniques that involve various types of multisensory cues. These specific techniques will be described in more complete detail in the next chapter. We think it wise to investigate these techniques or modifications of them with specific children with DAS to meet their very individual needs.

REMEDIATION SHOULD INCLUDE THE MANIPULATION OF PROSODIC FEATURES AS AN INTEGRAL PART OF THE TOTAL REMEDIAL PROGRAM. The use of rhythm, intonation, and stress facilitates the motor sequencing needed for speech production. Activities such as rhyming, singing, talking, or singing paired with arm and/or leg movement, stair-climbing, foot-tapping, finger-tapping, arm-swinging, beating time, clapping, whole body movements, squeezing an object on each syllable of a word, and use of stress markers added to printed or written reading stimuli can be useful techniques to introduce rhythm, stress, or intonation. Use of differential stress or intonation patterns have been suggested as being helpful (Rosenbek, Hansen, Baughman, and Lemme, 1974; Yoss & Darley, 1974b;

Macaluso-Haynes, 1978; Weiss, Gordon, & Lillywhite, 1987; Marquardt, Dunn, & Davis, 1985; & Marquardt and Sussman, 1991).

We too have found that the above listed activities have facilitated remediation of prosodic features. Stress and intonation, including loudness and rate, constitute another aspect of human communication—that of prosody. As discussed in Chapter 2, children with DAS are often thought to have problems with the prosody, or melody, of their oral expressive messages. Prosody is important in the conveying of emotional and linguistic information about the speaker's message. As such, prosody contributes to the overall intelligibility of the speaker. Thus, we take the position that variation in prosodic aspects of communication should be incorporated into the treatment program for children with DAS, and that prosodic goals should begin as a part of the early stages of treatment with the child.

We may need to accommodate a variety of features in developing prosodic goals for a particular client. Recall that our research has indicated that children with DAS are not devoid of prosodics, but that they may use prosodics inappropriately or inaccurately. So, some children may need to learn to use intensity more appropriately, while others may need to focus on appropriate use of inflections or stress. Most children respond well to dealing with the emotional use of prosody—producing an utterance as if they were excited, sad, afraid, etc. The inflectional differences between declarative and interrogative forms can also be targeted. The response needs to be modeled by the clinician so that the model exhibits both the correct articulatory production as well as the desired prosodic pattern. Gradually the modeling is faded, so that a request for a particular emotive state or grammatic form will elicit the correct use of prosody. This can be incorporated into all levels of speech work, from the isolated sound level to one in which the child is dealing with more complex speech tasks. Certainly the syntactic use (interrogative versus declarative inflection) is easier to deal with when phrase or sentence contexts are being targeted, but it is also possible to deal with these even at the single phoneme or syllable level, particularly if the responses are imitated from models provided by the clinician.

We have found that some of our patients with severe DAS involvement are not capable of working *simultaneously* with articulatory and prosodic goals. These children seem to be unable to hold onto more than one aspect of oral communication at a time. In these situations we first strive for achievement of an initial articulation goal. When this first speech goal is established, we add the prosody goal to the initial "easier" articulation task, demanding accuracy for not only the articulation but the prosody as well. The articulation goals may advance, although the prosody goal may lag behind the articulation goals as the hierarchy of complexity is increased.

Hargrove, Roetzel, and Hoodin (1989), in a multiple baseline single-subject design study, demonstrated that prosodic skills were modifiable with treatment. Their research methodology used "contradiction training" where a child was asked a question that obviously reflected an error in the speaker's understanding with the expected correct response containing increased stress on the word needing correction. Grube, Spiegel, Buchhop, and Lloyd (1986) compared use of intonation training with phonological processes in two preschoolers with severe intelligibility problems. Their results indicated that improved intelligibility was facilitated more by the intonation features than by the subjects' training of phonological processes. The intonation patterns targeted in the study were declaratives, interrogatives, and exclamatives through the use of modeled imitation plus motor movement to teach the skill. Although neither of these studies used children with DAS as subjects, the research paradigms might also be adapted for use in a remedial setting with this population.

The literature dealing with prosodic remediation with children is limited. Minskoff (1980b) makes both assessment and treatment suggestions, including teaching of feeling (emotion) conveyed by a particular vocal inflection, role-playing, and the giving of conflicting cues. Robin, Klouda, and Hug (1991) also make specific treatment suggestions for prosodic difficulties in neurologically-impaired adults that may be adapted for use with children with DAS. Additional information on the grammatical use of prosody, which may be helpful in developing remedial goals, is provided by Wode (1980).

THE CLINICIAN SHOULD, IF NECESSARY, TEACH COMPENSATORY STRATEGIES. The nature of DAS involves an inherent difficulty in sequencing speech sounds. Helping a child with DAS to successfully achieve this sequencing is often a clinical challenge and may include the purposeful teaching of compensatory strategies.

A frequently used strategy involves manipulation of prosodic elements such as slowing the overall rate of speech and increasing use of pauses between syllables and/or words (Rosenbek, Hansen, Baughman, and Lemme, 1974; Yoss and Darley, 1974b; Macaluso-Haynes, 1978; Blakeley, 1983; Marquardt, Dunn, and Davis, 1985; Weiss, Gordon, and Lillywhite, 1987; Air, Wood, and Neils, 1989; and Marquardt and Sussman, 1991). More specific suggestions on slowing rate are provided by Blakeley (1983) and Weiss et al. (1987) who suggest vowel prolongation and inclusion of the schwa between elements of blends (epenthesis). The acceptability of some of these suggestions may be dependent on the dialectal characteristics of the environment in which the child communicates.

The maintenance of targeted, or intended, sound sequences will help facilitate overall intelligibility, even if the listener may also be aware of the compensatory factors. The compensation may contribute to an unusual or different quality to the speech production, but this inclusion may help assist in the successful inclusion and production of more speech sounds.

We are in agreement that compensatory strategies may be a necessary part of therapy with children exhibiting DAS. Often we find that the children themselves come to recognize the helpfulness of one or more strategies. However, we strongly urge that clinicians promote use of compensatory techniques only as long as they are necessary or in circumstances in which the child *must* use their very best possible speech skills. Hopefully the strategies can be dispensed with as the child achieves better oral control and improved speech production.

The inclusion of the last two principles (manipulation of prosodics in the remedial program and the overt teaching of compensatory strategies) may seem to be in conflict. We do not think this to be the case. Rather we regard the compensatory strategies to be a phase or stage of remediation that facilitates a child's progress. Implementation of the strategies may give the child time to accurately make the desired movement sequences. When it is obvious that the compensation is no longer needed, we encourage clinicians to proceed with goal development which emphasizes typical use of rate, stress, etc.

THE CLINICIAN MUST PROVIDE SUCCESSFUL EXPERIENCES. Remedial programs and the development of individual goals within the programs must be designed so that the child with DAS appreciates their minute successes, the successes which direct the child to long-term goals. It seems that children with DAS have often learned through their remedial experiences to expect communication failure. Thus, often our first steps in remediation are to encourage the child to attempt speech activities, to not fear the possibility of failure, and to be willing to take risks with their speech.

Success can most easily be accomplished if the program begins at a level where the child can succeed. Sometimes the goals are skills that may be prerequisite to speech, such as imitating body or facial movements preparatory to imitating speech movements.

Reinforcement is important in the intervention provided to children with DAS. Reinforcement may be given both in verbal and token/tangible form and gives the child feedback on attempts at a speech target. Later, reductions in the percent of reinforcement help to maintain and establish the new speech behavior. As Lohr (1978) states: "Familiar tasks will require less frequent and tangible rewards; new and more difficult tasks will require more frequent and tangible rewards" (p. 5). Clinicians need to explore what particular reinforcers motivate each client and then use this to help the children acquire and establish the targeted speech behavior.

All children need success. Children with DAS specifically need success with speech goals targeted to help them realize that they are capable of making changes in their speech and to help them remain motivated, and cooperative clients through the long and slow remedial process which most probably awaits them.

CHAPTER 8

Remediation:
Specific Remedial Techniques

The literature contains a number of techniques or programs that were designed for remediation of DAS, or were developed for other communication disorders or populations and have been, or could be, adapted for use with children exhibiting DAS. The techniques do, or could, address varying aspects of the DAS disorder—some are designed to elicit or evoke phonemes when the child is unable to produce the phoneme after traditional and customary auditory and visual stimulation. Other techniques address the sequencing problems that are at the heart of the disorder, while others might facilitate better use of prosody. As long as the techniques used are compatible with a basic motor-programming framework, we think that there needs to be a willingness on the part of clinicians to insert or adapt a variety of specific therapy approaches to facilitate the progress of the individual child.

Techniques need to be reviewed individually to explore their potential contribution to remediation with DAS clients. When available in the literature, we present the theoretical basis and goal(s) for each approach, a description of the program, and a summary of available efficacy research. In addition, we indicate whether the technique is designed to be used for eliciting phonemes and/or used to address the speech sequencing problems of children with DAS. Readers may find reviews by Jaffe (1984, 1989), Pannbacker (1988), and Thompson (1988) to be helpful as well.

Multisensory and Tactile Cuing Techniques

A variety of techniques have been tried and suggested to provide successful cuing techniques. These techniques differ in the type of stimulation provided to teach and/or reinforce the child's production of movements necessary for sound production.

Moto-Kinesthetic Speech Training Method

Stinchfield and Young first described techniques in a 1938 text that were later called moto-kinesthetic by Young and (Stinchfield) Hawk (1955). The technique is based on the premise that

> the teacher visualizes the use to which the air current is to be put for each sound, and by direct stimulation, helps the muscular activity . . . to function correctly. . . . In the use of this method, another sense, the kinesthetic, is added as well as the tactile, to the use of visual and the auditory, thus associating the idea, the visual concept, the sound, and the feeling of the movements in sequence, all in one learning process. (Young and Hawk, 1955, p. 10)

When using this method the "teacher" or "trainer" directs muscular activity via a "standard stimulation" that "tends" to produce each phoneme. The teacher first analyses the changes needed in the air current to produce the sounds under the premise that action, or actions, of muscles upon the air current within the "upper passageways", in part, cause the speech sound to be produced. The location, direction, and form of speech movements are determined. The tactile stimulations identify the location of muscle function involved in speech production, while the kinesthetic aspect of the method comes into play as the child acquires the feeling of the movement direction. The teacher also provides an auditory stimulation for the targeted phoneme, or phoneme sequence, thus the child associates an auditory pattern with the feel of the movement sequences. An earlier description of a similar technique may have been made by Hadden, who reported in 1891 that when teaching Charles M. to speak "it was often necessary actually to adjust the part by the fingers or by forceps" (p.98). The moto-kinesthetic method, initially developed to assist "children with delayed or defective speech," deals with both elicitation of isolated phonemes as well as sequencing phonemes into words. Vowels and consonants are both addressed.

Young and (Stinchfield) Hawk (1955) stated that the goals for working specifically with vowels are that the exact sound be achieved and that continuity of the sound be maintained. The main stimulations for vowels are elevating or lowering the jaw, movement of the tongue, and movement of the lips so that the "air space within the mouth may be of definite shape and proportions" (p. 23). Young and Hawk stress the importance of vowels in the production of sound sequences.

In both editions of their text, the authors (Stinchfield & Young, 1938; Young & (Stinchfield) Hawk, 1955) provide descriptions of the stimulations the teacher or trainer needs to make in order to successfully elicit the individual sound or word pattern. Photographs of the positions are also included and may be helpful to the reader. In addition, Weiss, Gordon, and Lillywhite (1987) provide a summary of written descriptions of the moto-kinesthetic stimulations in their text.

Sara Stinchfield Hawk (1938, 1955) provides information regarding a research project she conducted. Improvement on speech scores was found following speech training. Presumably, the technique developed by Young and (Stinchfield) Hawk was used with some, if not all, of the 100 subjects. The efficacy of the remedial technique itself was not reported.

The moto-kinesthetic technique is one which the present authors have not used, and therefore, we cannot address our impressions of its effectiveness with children with DAS. The method may be helpful in assisting a child achieve the articulator placements necessary for isolated phoneme productions. Such placements are sometimes elusive, especially to those with severe DAS. However, the child would need to be tolerant of the manipulation of facial structures. Some children are tactically defensive, as reported by Dabul (1971), and for them this technique would be inappropriate. Further, this is a technique in which speech-language pathologists must receive direct training from an individual knowledgeable in its use, and such individuals seem now to be few in number. As Stinchfield and Young (1938) state: "It is not easy to describe the method, nor to show it in still pictures" (p. 96), also underscoring the need for a form of traineeship to develop proficiency with the technique. The scarcity of trained mentors may forecast the demise of the method before it has the opportunity to be fully evaluated for its effectiveness using research methodologies.

Association Method

McGinnis, Kleffner, and Goldstein (1956) published an article about a specific technique called the *Association Method* for teaching aphasic children. McGinnis later expanded this information in a text published in 1963 which she titled Aphasic Children. (This book was reprinted in 1988 as the second part of a classic text, *Teaching Aphasic Children*). Included in the subcategories of childhood aphasia was a group called *motor aphasics* whose communication difficulties were described and who exhibited characteristics we consider consistent with DAS. Aram and Nation (1982) note that the method has been adapted by clinicians in their work with children exhibiting DAS. McGinnis (1963) developed the Association Method because it provided "a close association of the essential processes of learning, i.e., attention, retention, and recall" (p. 59). Especially important is the association of the written form of the sounds with their articulation, as well as the child's skill in analyzing and monitoring the speech productions that are being taught.

According to the McGinnis (1963) text, the method emphasizes the movements of precisely articulated sounds so that the child establishes a kinesthetic sense of the actual movement. The child is thought to be learning by visual, auditory, and kinesthetic impression, which facilitates the retention and recall of the sounds or words when stimulated by its written form, a picture, or the actual object.

The Association Method is a formal, structured program, but McGinnis (1963) states 4 years is a good age at which to initiate work with the method. The method itself consists of a vertical program (a sequence of items comprising the total curriculum) which includes a number of steps within three units carried out during a horizontal, or daily, program. The *First Unit of Language* targets the goal of acquisition of 50 nouns. The *Second* and *Third Units of Language* include work with syntax and vocabulary development while the articulation skills are dealt with through *Correlative Programs.*

We are unaware of any research addressing the efficacy of the Association Method. Neither have we used the technique ourselves with our clients exhibiting DAS. As described by McGinnis, it is a method that needs specific training to execute.

Sensory-Motor (McDonald) Approach

The Sensory-Motor Approach was developed by Eugene McDonald and published in 1964. The Approach was developed for individuals with articulation problems and is "designed to bring about greater specificity in the sequences of the overlapping ballistic movements through which speech sounds are produced" (p. 135). The program does not address the elicitation of phonemes but rather deals with sequential movements.

The first objective of the approach is "to heighten the child's responsiveness to the patterns of auditory, proprioceptive, and tactile sensations associated with the overlapping ballistic movements of articulation" (p. 138). Auditory models are provided, which the child is asked to imitate and then describe in terms of tactile and movement sensations. The movements progress from simple to complex with a variety of stress patterns so the performance of overlapping movements is emphasized. This is done initially with reduplicated bisyllables (CVCV), then with varying stress patterns during reduplicated bisyllables. Later syllable combinations are used where the vowel and/or consonants vary (CV_1CV_2, C_1VC_2V, $C_1V_1C_2V_2$). Finally, trisyllables are developed and are produced with varying stress patterns. McDonald suggests starting with combinations where large shifts of movement are needed and later requiring smaller movement shifts within the combinations in the trisyllables. Initially, phonemes already evident in the child's repertoire should be used in development of remedial stimuli, although as progress is made in learning to listen, remembering entire sequences, and describing the direction of movement, errored sounds should be included in the trisyllables. During this objective "correct articulation should be reinforced through repetition" (p. 142).

The second objective is "to reinforce the child's articulation of his error sound" (p. 142). Guidelines are provided to help the clinician decide which sound should be reinforced, including selecting a phoneme that is correct in at least one context of the *Deep Test of Articulation* (McDonald, 1964). The next stage of the objective is to use a context in which the errored sound is correctly articulated to reinforce correct sensory-motor patterns. An example is provided in which a child mis-articulates /s/ except when it is preceded by /tʃ/ and followed by an /ɚ/ vowel, as in the sequence /watʃ sʌn/ or "watchsun." This sensory-motor pattern is strengthened by various production procedures involving slowed movements, various stress patterns, use of written stimuli, and inclusion of the sequence into meaningful sentences.

The third objective is "to facilitate the correct articulation of the sound in systematically varied phonetic contexts" (p. 146). This is accomplished by changing vowels following the targeted phoneme, both in spoken and written formats, and practicing the expanded group of correctly produced contexts into additional word combinations that can then be placed in sentences and produced with a variety of stress patterns.

We have not found efficacy studies using this approach in remediation with children presenting DAS. However, in a retrospective review of 10 semesters of remediation conducted with a child exhibiting DAS, Marquardt and Sussman (1991) stated that use of the McDonald sensory-motor drill "helped to establish seven sounds in medial position and to stabilize a number of transitions from varying consonants" (p. 385).

Rosenbek and Wertz (1972) suggested that this remedial approach would be appropriate for young children with DAS. From our motor-programming perspective, the techniques associated with at least the first objective of McDonald's Sensory-Motor approach may well be helpful to children with DAS. This is because of the type of structuring needed with which to develop appropriate stimuli, and the approach's emphasis on slow increments in difficulty level, numerous repetitions of the stimuli, and inclusion of various prosodic features.

Prompts for Restructuring Oral Muscular Phonetic Targets (PROMPT)

The Prompts for Restructuring Oral Muscular Phonetic Targets (PROMPT) system, developed by Deborah Chumpelik (1984), is a method of treatment for DAS that focuses on the "impaired abilities to organize and produce volitional speech sounds and sequences" (p. 139). The system is organized so that DAS is treated as a movement disorder, with the treatment focusing on the programming aspects of motor control. Speech production is handled by having a target position or sequence imposed on the child. Chumpelik said that, unlike other treatment programs, PROMPT does not use imitation or perceptual comparisons to organize or control movements. Instead, targets are used to aid the child in making speech productions, with tactile and kinesthetic prompts being imposed on the child to ensure that feedback is present. Further, she indicated that the system "imposes control on the articulators by providing tactile and kinesthetic (closed-loop) feedback, while guiding the structures toward sequential, feed-forward (open-loop) programming. The general effect is one of reducing inadequate feedback and providing correct movement sequences in order to help establish 'normal' speech-motor production" (p. 144).

The system is described as a tactile-based treatment method where different external prompts are given to the muscles of the face and under the chin, as well as to the structures associated with voicing, nasality, and jaw opening. Chumpelik (1984) states that the timing of each prompt given by the clinician to the child is crucial, especially when used during phrase and sentence production. Prompts were developed for all English phonemes, and all involve the following: (1) place of contact, (2) degree of jaw closure, (3) manner or features (duration, continuancy, movement, fusion, lateralization, labialization) important to production, (4) the muscles used in specific phoneme productions, (5) the amount of tension needed by the specific muscles and muscle groups, (6) timing, and (7) stressing patterns. The system was developed to elicit phonemes, but the prompts can also be used serially so that sequential speech movements can be facilitated whether they are in a blend or within words or phrases.

Chumpelik (1984) cites a study she conducted comparing the PROMPT system with a traditional audiovisual technique. The specific data were not reported, but "results indicated that for more difficult targets—some vowels, consonants with tension, and timing factors—the PROMPT system was the only way to produce change" (p. 150). We have been unable to find any efficacy research using the PROMPT system with children exhibiting DAS.

We have not used this system in our own work with children presenting DAS. A problem with it, and with many of the other such tactile-based cuing techniques, may be that some clinicians feel uncomfortable with the sustained touching of their clients. Also, some children are touch defensive and may react very negatively to this type of remediation for this reason. When evaluating the appropriateness of this type of system, the client's tolerance for such touching needs to be a top consideration. In addition, it appears that this may be a technique where specialized training is necessary in order to use it successfully and in a consistent manner.

Touch-Cue Method

Bashir, Grahamjones, and Bostwick (1984) describe a Touch-Cue method of remediation with children exhibiting DAS. It is reported to be based on the assumption that the "child has difficulty in firmly establishing and integrating voluntary oral motor movements necessary for purposes of speech sound production. In addition, the child experiences difficulties in incorporating these motor patterns into synergies of movement necessary for the production of connected speech" (p. 128). The developers of the method stress that it is one that addresses speech-sound *sequencing,* and is not a "speech-sound *teaching*" program.

The program is described as a direct and systematic approach to the articulation learning of eight phonemes for which cues have been developed, which moves through three discrete stages. As implied by the name of the approach, touch cues are administered by the clinician, or in some instances, the client themselves, to the lower face or neck for the following phonemes: /b/, /d/, /g/, /s/, /f/, /n/, /ʃ/, and /l/. The "topographic indicators" (cues) are given simultaneously with auditory and visual cues during the initial phase of therapy. Cues for additional phonemes may be developed by the clinician to meet the specific needs of the child but must be consistent.

The three stages incorporated in the method are described with a series of goals for each stage being prescribed. The phonemes are also recommended to be addressed in a specific order that is reflected in the listing presented in the previous paragraph. Stage I is possible only if a child is capable of producing a phoneme in isolation and involves a series of nonsense syllable drills to facilitate the teaching of the topographic cues, improving articulatory sequencing, and developing accurate self-monitoring of productions. The chained repetition drills with these specific phonemes are to continue until the criterion of 95% correct in 20 trials (19/20) is achieved. Stage II consists of drills that place the previously learned sequential movements into monosyllabic words using the CVC configuration, as well as into polysyllabic words. The stimulus lists contain both real and nonsense words that emphasize contrasts in place, manner, and voicing aspects of productions. The use of auditory, visual, and tactile cues is manipulated and faded throughout Stage II, with the introduction of graphic or picture stimuli. The 95% criterion for success is maintained. The goal for Stage III is for the child with DAS to apply the sequencing and self-monitoring skills to productions of controlled multiword utterances and then in spontaneous speech. The program is considered completed when, in spontaneous speech, the child's speech is intelligible all of the time and when the child "can monitor and subsequently, self-correct speech most of the time" (Bashir et al., 1984, p. 136).

There is no efficacy information provided concerning the Touch-Cue remedial approach. It is highly systematic and involves the intensive drills that we consider important to remedial success with children exhibiting DAS. The number of phonemes for which the cues have been developed is limited, however, the drawings of the cues seem clear. The clinician is encouraged to develop cues other than these eight. Thus, the system may be more easily used without direct training than are other systems using tactile cues. The program also allows for the client to be taught to use the cues to help themselves, one possible solution to a client who is touch defensive. However, many children with DAS do not have sufficient fine motor skills of the hands to execute the cues and sufficient awareness of the intended phoneme targets to know when to apply them during the drills.

Rood Technique

Margaret Rood published an article in 1954 that described an approach to physical and occupational therapy with individuals exhibiting cerebral palsy. Her original publication, along with Stockmeyer's (1967) later interpretation of the technique, detail the theory of neuromuscular dysfunction on which the approach is based. The reader is referred to the original sources for a full explanation of the techniques's theoretical framework.

Haynes (1985) suggests the use of Rood's technique to increase orosensory perceptual awareness.

> If deficits in orosensory awareness are identified through careful diagnostic procedures, attempts can then be made to increase the patient's awareness of the orosensory mechanism by bombarding it with multisensory stimuli. Since tactile stimulation reportedly has a facilitating effect on the pyramidal tract, which in turn, is responsible for more skills or planned motion, it would then appear reasonable to use tactile stimulation to improve the patient's orosensitivity and awareness. (p. 263)

Haynes cited techniques such as icing, brushing, rubbing, or touching oral structures with toothbrushes. Various textures such as cotton and sandpaper are suggested for application to the child's upper lip, tongue, palate, and buccal area to provide additional stimulation. Also suggested are application of "deep pressure" and "resistance" techniques. Haynes also stated that there is a close relationship between taste and smell and so suggested olfactory stimulation with ammonia and (rubbing) alcohol, as well as taste stimulation with the use of "unpleasant or bitter foods," suggesting lemon and grapefruit. She further suggested that "prolonged" stimulation, which could be used at home with the child, would be the eating of "candy of various shapes, sizes, and textures."

We are not aware of any research testing the efficacy of these techniques. We question the application of such techniques to treatment of speech sound disorders. Rood (1954) and Stockmeyer (1967) reported the techniques as helpful in their clinical work with children with cerebral palsy and adults with hemiplegia in eliciting gross motor movement and postures. We suspect that the techniques might be worthy of consideration when attempts are made to establish the positioning of the articulators for sound production after other elicitation techniques have failed. If collaborating with a physical therapist and/or an occupational therapist, consultation in treatment of the child before using the techniques would assure consistency of management.

Speech Facilitation

Speech Facilitation was developed by Vaughn and Clark (1979) in an attempt to clarify and expand upon explanations of the extraoral stimulations involved with Young and Hawk's (1955) moto-kinesthetic technique and to describe the development and use of phonodental guides. It was reported to be developed for individuals with articulation disorders, including preschool and primary school children, the deaf, individuals with mental retardation, and persons with neurologically based articulation problems. Speech Facilitation involves the combined use of both extraoral manipulation and intraoral stimulation to facilitate the production of both consonants and vowels. The intraoral stimulations are provided by phonodental guides that purport to facilitate tongue placement, while the extraoral manipulations purport to facilitate the movement involved in a phoneme elicitation. Vaughn and Clark (1979) state that the technique can be used as the primary or supplementary one within a total intervention program.

The application of extraoral stimulations are guided by four principles: (1) a rapport must be established between the "stimulator" (clinician) and "respondent" (client); (2) the position and movement for each phoneme is taught; (3) timing, rate, pressure, duration, and stress are used; and (4) auditory and visual sensory stimuli may be added to or deleted from the stimulation protocol. The extraoral stimulations consist of manipulation models of a lips format with numbered points, a finger and hand format, and a face format with numbered points. The finger and hand format involves placing a finger on the side of the nose to cue nasalization, touching the larynx with a finger to cue phonation, and pressing the palm of one hand below the client's rib cage to cue breath expiration, with the amount of hand pressure used to activate sudden or gradual expiration. The extraoral stimulations or manipulations for each consonant and vowel phoneme are described in Vaughn and Clark's (1979) text.

The intraoral stimulation is provided by six types of phonodental guides: (1) oral acrylic modifiers, (2) orthodontic wire guides, (3) denture guides, (4) dental floss guides (knotted and stretched), (5) various types of stemmed wire guides, and (6) cue sticks. Vaughn and Clark (1979) described the availability or preparation of each guide, as well as their use in eliciting phonemes.

No work regarding efficacy is reported by Vaughn and Clark (1979). The stimulations would seem most appropriate for the elicitation of phonemes. The extraoral stimulations provide yet another technique involving tactile-types of cue systems. While we have previously cautioned about negative aspects of remediation approaches based on touch, Vaughn and Clark note that some persons enjoy being touched and suggest that this may offer reassurance to some clients, while promoting rapport between the clinician and client. We also have some reservations, in this day and age, about any remedial program such as this that requires the clinician to touch any part of the body other than the face and neck area because the intent may be misinterpreted.

The "phonodental guides" used for intraoral stimulation are unique. However, we suggest consideration of these only when less invasive techniques have been shown to fail with a particular client exhibiting DAS. It is possible that use of the guides could scrape or puncture mouth tissue with resultant blood. Thus, as a precaution, we urge consideration of appropriate protective techniques to be used by the clinician. The technique, like so many others, probably needs instruction from the master-clinicians who developed them or "guidance from a clinician experienced in the technique" (p. ix) in order for the manipulation to be executed appropriately and for the guides to be used correctly. Vaughn and Clark (1979) state "the effectiveness of the stimulations is usually proportional to the skill of the clinician" (p. ix).

Gestural Cuing Techniques

A variety of remediation techniques have incorporated manually presented cuing to suggest or elicit oral responses from the child.

Signed Target Phoneme Therapy (STP)

Shelton and Graves (1985) described a remedial program they called Signed Target Phoneme Therapy (STP) which was developed for a 5-year-old child with DAS. The approach was based on the thought that visual memory and an "internalized visual stimulus" could assist a child with DAS in recalling what articulatory gestures to make.

The visual cues of STP are based on the hand shapes from the American Manual Alphabet and are executed simultaneously with an auditory model of the target sound. Only the *targeted* phoneme(s), not all phonemes, in a stimulus are cued gesturally by the clinician. The child is not required to produce the cue during his or her oral response, but the authors of the method indicate that this might be an advantageous facilitator. The approach does not address actual acquisition or teaching of phonemes but may facilitate sequencing of phonemes. STP was designed to be added to traditional therapy methods.

The authors of the technique, Shelton and Graves (1985), present a case review of a 5-year-old child with DAS with whom STP was used to facilitate correct production. Two clinicians alternated in conducting the traditional intervention with the initial /s/ phoneme. One clinician incorporated STP and the other did not. The child was reported to have reached criterion "more quickly in fewer sessions" using STP, although no data are provided to support the statement. Shelton and Graves suggest that further documentation is needed, however.

The description of the program implies that both consonants and vowels are dealt with in the technique, although examples include only consonants. There is an inherent restriction since one hand shape per letter has been developed, and a single letter (grapheme) can represent several vowel sounds.

We think that the system may be helpful to some children, particularly those who appear to benefit from multi-modality stimuli. We encourage researchers to demonstrate its efficacy. Along those lines, we encourage clinicians who use the technique to provide visual cues to their clients with DAS and to encourage the child to use the cues as well. However, we must remember that children with DAS may also exhibit limb apraxias. As a result, the child may be unable to produce the gestures, or modification of the gestures may need to be accepted. Our clinical hunch suggests that this system, if not used in its entirety, may have applicability for an individual child demonstrating problems with specific unique phoneme(s).

Adapted Cuing Technique (ACT)

The Adapted Cuing Technique (ACT) was developed for the treatment of dyspraxia by Klick (1985) and consists of manually presented visual cues "created to accompany orally presented speech" (p. 256). The technique purports to enhance oral stimuli and to increase the frequency of correct responses for both consonants and vowels on the part of the client, particularly during sequential speech movements.

No theoretical basis for the actual development of the specific cuing technique is provided, although literature suggesting use of the visual modality and remedial emphasis on sequential articulatory movement in DAS is noted by the technique's originator.

Klick's descriptions of her technique includes the following:

ACT reflects the shapes of the oral cavity and movements required during speech production. Patterns of articulatory movement and the manner of production of sounds are made visible by motions of the clinician's hand. In general the clinician's hand is held near his/her face and is in motion while the clinician says the word or phrase to be repeated by the client. In cuing place of production, the trajectory of the tongue, rather than its static placement, is represented . . . . Hand motions also cue manner changes by depicting airflow release. Movements of the hand within its overall motion cue two sound classes, stops and continuants . . . . Finger movements signal specific speech sounds . . . held in configurations loosely based on those of the manual alphabet for the deaf . . . Cuing vowels is an essential part of ACT. (pp. 256–257)

Klick (1985) stated that, when using ACT, vowels are cued along two dimensions, which are the place of articulation and the degree of jaw closure. "All vowels are signaled by variations of the letter c handshape. The hand is held with the fingers pointing toward the cheek. Jaw closure is represented by the degree of closure between the fingers and thumb of the c handshape. Moving the hand toward the front, middle, or back of the oral tract cues placement" (p. 257).

Klick (1985) also provided a case study of a *dyspraxic* 5½-year-old girl with whom the technique was successful. After 3 months of remediation using the technique, oral communication skills were judged to have improved. This was documented by the inclusion of several carrier phrases and 12 single words that could be functionally produced. After an additional 3 months of treatment Klick noted that the client had begun to produce novel utterances. As well, Klick also cited parental reports of increased intelligibility and verbal output in the home setting.

ACT, as with the several other manual/gestural systems that have been presented in this chapter, seems able to provide the child with DAS additional visual stimulation which may facilitate production and sequencing of phonemes. The technique appears to be one that could be incorporated within motor-programming approaches to DAS treatment. Klick (1985) notes that the client occasionally self-cued; we question if the usefulness of the technique could not be expanded to include this additional gestural-motor stimulation. As Klick notes, the technique uses the gestures of the manual alphabet, already systemized and widely used by speech and hearing professionals in their work with the hearing impaired. Thus, this aspect of ACT would be in place for many clinicians who might want to consider its use with their clients with DAS. However, we found the written descriptions of the technique somewhat difficult to understand; the usefulness of the technique may be limited to a few clinicians because of the need to learn it from an individual who knows and uses it.

Cued Speech

Cued Speech was developed by Cornett (1972) at Gallaudet College for lipreading use by the deaf. The system purports to differentiate each speech sound with a set of 12 cues: eight hand shapes and four basic hand positions, which, when used in combination, result in a total of 32 possible cues. Each of the hand shapes represents three or four consonants from different viseme groups, that are distinguishable from each other in lipreading contexts. Each of the hand positions involves four locations about the face and represent two or three vowels, also from different groups of phonemes which look the same during lipreading. The goal of Cued Speech is to facilitate the lipreading of words which are homophenous or appear the same when only visual cues during word production are available such as the words "pop," "Bob," and "Mom".

Cornett (personal correspondence) proposed to the authors that Cued Speech might facilitate sequencing of articulatory movements by children with DAS. Sequencing would be facilitated by the clinician providing a motor (cuing) sequence which the child could duplicate and associate with speech production, initially element by element and then sequentially.

Gallaudet University provides several studies in which Cued Speech was reported to be successfully used with deaf children and adolescents. We are not aware of any studies that have used this technique with children with normal hearing to facilitate speech production or sequencing.

If a clinician is familiar with the Cued Speech system and is able to use it with children with hearing impairments, its use with clients exhibiting DAS could also be explored. Learning the individual cues involved with Cued Speech would appear easy to do and might provide assistance to the clinicians of a child exhibiting DAS who is dealing with phoneme elicitation/evocation. However, as Davis and Hardick (1981) point out, combining the cues into sequences requires extensive practice, thus perhaps reducing the system's usefulness for this aspect of remediation.

We have not employed this system in our work with clients presenting DAS. While it may be useful, the system seems more cumbersome to learn and execute than other manual systems. The original purpose was to reduce visual confusion in lipreading, but information differentiating phonemes that look alike during production has not been demonstrated to be useful to a child with DAS, and it is perhaps not the most salient information to assist children with DAS in producing a phoneme or to sequence them correctly. Further, Cued Speech is not as extensively used as are other manual/gestural systems, either by speech-language

pathologists or by other educators, again reducing its potential helpfulness to the child with DAS simply because fewer people in their environment would be facile in using it for production assistance. As with the
other manual systems, we think that the child should also be taught
to use the system for self-cuing purposes, allowing for additional
kinesthesthic feedback, although the presence of limb apraxia may negate
or restrict its successful use by the child with DAS.

Visual Phonics

Visual Phonics (International Communication Learning Institute, 1981)
is described as a visual and kinesthetic method using a system of hand
signs and written symbols developed to help the deaf learn to speak and
read. It would be difficult to learn the hand signs without the opportunity
to view the training tape, as the hand signs are not static and the required
movements are not indicated by the written symbols. Forty-five signs/
sounds are tested and subsequently taught. The production of the sounds
progresses from production in isolation to production in words and then
to production in sentences. Principles of co-articulation are not addressed.
It is our impression that the relationships between the configuration of
the hand shape, the written symbol, and the grapheme are in many
instances quite abstract. The procedures stress that the child must make
the hand sign while he or she attempts to say the sound. The demonstra-
tion tape admits that it may be difficult for a child to achieve the hand
positions. Furthermore, we think, the production of "k," "q," "x," and
"c" are difficult to differentiate, and appear to address reading, not speech
production, goals.

The end result of the original purpose of Visual Phonics was for the
child to read sounds, progress to words, and move on to sentences. The
procedure may be of some use for children with DAS, but we are unaware
of any but anecdotal comments about efficacy with any population. We
question the practical approach of using a system dedicated to teaching
reading.

Jordan's Gestures

We recognize that there is a need for techniques beyond modeling for
informing the child about a phoneme's contact points and manner of production. To this end, Jordan (1988, 1991) developed a system of gestures
to give an adult with apraxia of speech information about the configuration of the oral cavity. This included information about the point of con-
striction within the oral cavity necessary for production of the target
consonant sound, whether movement of the structures is necessary, and
whether movement of the vocal folds accompanies production of the pho-

neme. Figure 8.1 illustrates the gestures developed for the phonemes /m/, /p/, and /b/.

Jordan's gestures (1988) were particularly effective with the reported adult patient because he was able to use the gestures for self-cuing and retained use of them until the speech postures became automatic. The system has been used in its entirety with one other adult patient with equal success.

We have used the gestures with children with DAS attending our intensive summer residential program to teach production of problematic phonemes. These gestures were incorporated within a motor-programming approach to remediation. Because of time constraints and because other approaches had been successful with selected phonemes,

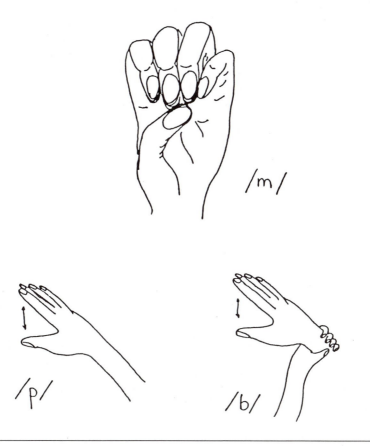

FIGURE 8.1. Jordan's Gestures for the /m/, /p/, and /b/ phonemes. *Note.* From "Gestures for cuing phonemes in verbal apraxia: A case study" by L. S. Jordan, 1988. Paper presented at the annual meeting of the American Speech-Language-Hearing Association, Boston. Reprinted by permission of the author.

we did not judge it practical, or necessary, to teach the entire set of gestures to any of the children. In addition, the children were encouraged to produce the gestures for self-cuing purposes.

A single subject multiple baseline design was used to obtain data from the children with whom we have incorporated use of Jordan's Gestures (Hall & Jordan, 1992). As might be expected with children with DAS, variable day to day results were recorded. However, results indicated idiosyncratic improvements for all. For instance, one child responded well to the differentiating gesture for voice/voiceless cognates. Another responded well to incorporation of the medial /θ/ and later to the /r/ in blends. A third child found the /s/ gesture helpful with /s/-blends, although earlier in the summer he did not seem to find the gesture helpful with singleton /s/.

In summary, it appears that adults and children find the concrete representations of the oral cavity configurations helpful in phoneme production. However, Jordan's Gestures, like other gestural systems, need to be further scrutinized for the efficacy of the procedure. The learning of the system is fairly straightforward and has been easily acquired by clinicians associated with our clinic, as well as the children with DAS who were taught selected gestures. However, before initiating the system with a child exhibiting DAS, the presence of limb apraxia must be assessed.

Miscellaneous Techniques

A variety of other techniques have been used in the remediation of children with DAS. No single descriptive term applies to these techniques. However, since they may be useful with a given child with DAS, we include them here.

Melodic Intonation Therapy (MIT)

Melodic Intonation Therapy (MIT), a therapy technique developed by Albert, Sparks, and Helm (1973) and Sparks, Helm, and Albert (1974), has been suggested for use with children with DAS. The procedure was developed for use with adult aphasic patients who have good comprehension but very limited verbal output. Supposedly, it takes advantage of emphasizing the melodic pattern of a phrase or sentence and requires the patient to accompany the clinician's model of tapping out the rhythm and intoning the words of the phrase or sentence. This purports to foster recovery/use of language. In the adult population, the use of this technique, while it resulted in more fluent production of the language, also resulted in enhanced accuracy of motor programming of speech production.

Use of the MIT technique with children exhibiting DAS has been reported to improve articulatory accuracy and prosodic features in one 10-year-old (Doszak, McNeil, & Jancosek, 1981) and articulation and sequencing abilities in two 7- and 8-year-olds (Helfrich-Miller, 1984). Krauss and Galloway (1982) and Schumacher, McNeil, Vetter, and Yoder (1984) have documented the efficacy of MIT in the treatment of children with developmental apraxia of speech. Hyland and McNeil (1987) have demonstrated usefulness of the technique with a developmentally apraxic adult.

Three elements of spoken prosody are recognized in MIT. The melodic line, or variation of pitch, in a spoken phrase or sentence using a vocal range of 3-4 whole notes is the element from which the strategy received its name. Equally important are the elements of tempo and rhythm and the use of points of distinct stress within the phrase to create the spoken prosody. The clinician maintains control by hand tapping (holding the patient's left hand), which serves to cue the client's response. The clinician presents the model of the stimulus, which the aphasic attempts to imitate. The clinician fades first the presentation of the auditory, then the visual model until the client is performing in isolation.

Good candidates for MIT have "essentially normal" (Sparks & Deck, 1986, page 322) understanding and retention of spoken language. Except for occasional stereotypical utterances, they have only indistinct speech. The client has an acute awareness of errors and makes multiple efforts to correct them.

Helfrich-Miller (1984) adapted the MIT program for use with children 7 to 8 years old with a MLR of 3-4 words, poor repetition skills, and an attention span of 15-20 minutes. Signed English was substituted for the hand tapping that was developed for the adults, and the program progressed through three stages that increased output length and phonemic complexity and reduced reliance on the clinician and on intonation. We find it difficult to imagine that using signed English would not impose restrictions on tempo and rhythm.

As described by Sparks and Deck (1986, p. 322), seven principles are involved in MIT. They are:

1. Treatment proceeds through increments in length and difficulty of task.

2. Because the aphasic can seldom recall the specific characteristics of his errors on the target response, he is led back to the preceding response and then guided to a second attempt of the target response.

3. Repetition serves as the core of MIT but only repetition of familiar units.

4. Timing and latency are controlled to reduce perseveration or the onset of a series of failures resulting from
focal fatigue.

5. Meaningful materials are used to trigger recall of pre-
morbid language skills, but a wide variety are used so
as to avoid practice effect.

6. Vigilance must be exercised over the clinician's own
verbal behavior so as not to disrupt the progression of
the treatment without direct purpose.

7. Treatment sessions are scheduled as intensively as
schedules and resources allow.

Principles 2, 3, and 5 imply to us that the client (aphasic) has some
knowledge of what the goal and production is or would have been. We
have some concerns about assuming that the child with DAS has such
insight or foreknowledge of goals. Although the child with DAS frequently
appears to be aware of communication failure, we do not believe that
he or she is aware of specific characteristics that are in error. With reservations about the child's lack of experience and self-knowledge, the principles, as stated above, are consistent with what we consider to be good
programming with children with DAS.

Krauss and Galloway (1982) reflect that "some verbal output appears
to be essential for MIT to be effective" (p. 112). Many of the children
with whom we work, at least initially, have limited, if any, expressive
vocabularies. Thus, we have not been motivated to try this treatment with
children. It appears to us to be imperative that characteristics of children
with DAS, who will be good candidates for melodic intonation therapy,
need to be identified.

The original authors of MIT recommended that no other language
therapy program be used concurrently with it, theorizing that "disin-
hibition of the right hemisphere might be delayed if intoning as well as
normal speech prosody are demanded" (Sparks & Deck, 1986, p. 331).
Concomitant programs, whether provided by a speech-language pathologist or some other individual involved with the child's care, need to
be scrupulously described. We cannot be so presumptuous as to assume
that we are the only communicative influence in a child's life, but we
must at least be able to describe the impact of other contacts. We are
not at ease eliminating other efforts that might provide the child with
successful communicative experiences. Goals such as improving vocabulary size or improving syntactic abilities appear to be appropriate goals
that might offer increased success in communication.

Our reservations about limited evidence of efficacy are applicable
to this technique. Identification of such skills as auditory pattern recogni-

tion may be relevant. The level of initial verbal output necessary for some success to be possible also needs to be determined.

Multiple Phonemic (Multi-Phonemic) Approach

The Multiple Phonemic Approach to remediation was developed during what some would call the "Operant Era" in speech-language pathology. Originally presented by Bradley and McCabe (1971), description of the technique was followed by a journal article published by McCabe and Bradley (1975) and a book chapter by Bradley (1989). The method was intended to provide intensive remediation programming for clients exhibiting six or more articulatory errors. The targeted population for which the approach was originally intended was children with repaired cleft palate and other types of maxio-facial anomalies. More recently, the approach was cited as one of several used with a child exhibiting DAS who was presented in a case study format by Davis, Marquardt, and Sussman (1985) and by Marquardt and Sussman (1991).

The rationale for the development of the Multi-Phonemic Approach was to deal with all of an individual's errored consonantal phonemes during a remedial session. There is an operant orientation to the approach that systematizes the programming, data collection, and criterion levels, while maintaining the progression through the complexity levels of conventional articulation therapy. The approach is divided into three phases and each of the phases is then divided into steps.

As described by Bradley (1989), Phase I is the Establishment phase, with the goal that "the speaker should produce each consonant sound of English in response to a grapheme or phonetic symbol representing it" (p. 308). This is accomplished by stimulation of all phonemes, errored or not. Phonemes are stimulated in CV syllables (consonant and one neutral vowel) through a series of stimulations. Level C stimulation requires the greatest amount of structure via the use of auditory, visual, and phonemic placement stimuli; Level B uses auditory and visual stimuli; and Level A requires the least amount of structure with only visual (written) stimuli. To succeed in Phase I, the child must produce five consecutive accurate responses during one session or four of the five production attempts for two consecutive sessions, which "has the ultimate goal of using all error sounds accurately in conversational speech" (p. 310).

Phase II is the Transfer phase. This is accomplished through five steps that need to be documented for each session. The Phase II steps are syllable practice, words, phrases/sentences, reading/story, and conversation. All errored phonemes are targeted during each session with the probability that work on each phoneme would be conducted at a different complexity level. Criterion of 80%–90% is prescribed.

Phase III is the Maintenance phase with the goal "to maintain at least 90% whole-word accuracy in various speaking situations without support from therapy sessions or other external monitoring" (p. 315). An accuracy level of 95% is cited as the level typically maintained 3 months after the termination of remedial services.

McCabe and Bradley (1975) state that the clinician should focus on as many phonemes during an individual therapy session as time will allow. They also note that at each level of intervention, the client is at an appropriate production ability level since for each client work continues at a level until the stated criterion level is reached, at which time the difficulty level is advanced to the next step or phase. Further, they note that the approach's structure is flexible so the needs of each individual child can be met.

McCabe and Bradley (1975) report on data collected over a 3-year time period with 44 patients, 5 to 14 years of age. Pre- and Post-therapy formal test scores provided information on changes that had occurred in the articulation over 10 weeks (45-50 hours) of remediation. A significant difference was found to be present within the group of 44 patients at the word level between the two test administrations that assessed only specific target phonemes within the stimuli. It should be remembered that these results were constrained to word level due to the nature of the assessment instrument. The pre- and post-therapy results from a research-developed articulation protocol were also analyzed and found to be significant when whole-word accuracy was assessed. No information on changes in performance in contexts more difficult than single words was provided.

Davis, Marquardt, and Sussman (1985) and Marquardt and Sussman (1991) reported that the Multi-Phonemic Approach was used during the third and fourth semesters of the 10 semesters reviewed in their extensive case presentation of a single client who exhibited DAS. Their conclusion was that the approach was successful in the establishment of the initial productions of targeted phonemes in CV and VC sequences. Use of the approach was not reported beyond the syllable level.

The systematic nature of the technique has some appeal, although we have not used the approach with children with DAS. It forces a clinician to be very aware of the types of stimulation that a child needs in order to succeed in Phase I. The approach also has specific criteria that must be met before a task-level is advanced; Bradley (1989) states that the steps can be broken down into smaller increments should a child seem to need it. Our concern about the approach with children presenting DAS is that it conceptually requires a child to deal with many (all) errored phonemes during a single remedial session. This is a task that is beyond many of the children with DAS whom we see. However, there is a stage of remediation during which it may be helpful for a client with DAS to be required to make frequent changes in targets and to do so accurately. At the time when this is an appropriate goal, the approach would seem helpful. Phases II and III would likely need to be broken into much smaller targeted steps than are described by McCabe and Bradley (1975). The Multiple Phoneme Approach needs to be scrutinized by systematic study as to its efficacy with this special population of clients.

Instrumental Feedback

Technology is becoming an ally of the speech-language pathologist. Instrumentation is now available that can help the client visualize what is happening in their mouths during speech production. Instrumentation allows the client to see the spectral read-out of his/her production and match this with the visual read-out of the correct target, which is provided by the clinician or speech synthesis. Present technologies offer dynamic palatometry, which provides visual feedback of tongue and palate contacts during phoneme production; glossometry, which measures changes in the tongue height and shape during vowel production; and ultrasound, which provides visual feedback of tongue position and shape.

Hardcastle, MorganBarry, and Clark (1987) described the use of electropalatography (EPG) in the diagnostic process. Their four subjects showed lingual-palatal contact patterns that differed in "both spatial configuration and variability" (p. 171) from normal subjects. As a result of this work, the tentative diagnosis of *verbal dyspraxia* was made for two of the four subjects.

MorganBarry (1989) later reported the use of EPG within the remedial programming of four patients, including one of the subjects whom the earlier Hardcastle, MorganBarry, and Clark (1987) study had diagnosed as being dyspraxic. It was hypothesized that the visual feedback capabilities of the system would be helpful in acquisition of tongue positions. MorganBarry stressed that the use of EPG was incorporated into more conventional remedial programs. She further states that EPG was intended to supplement, not replace, more traditional approaches. The phonemes selected for EPG-assisted remediation were the /l/, with later progression to the alveolar contacts /t,d,n/. The results of the study stated that all four of the subjects responded in some measure to the visual feedback system. MorganBarry cautiously addressed the progress achieved by the child with dyspraxia, noting that he enjoyed working with the EPG system but "found it very difficult to monitor movements and to establish acceptable sounds into words and phrases; his inability to sequence sounds, and faulty habits of articulatory movement hindered improvement in this area" (p.90).

The MorganBarry (1989) article shares some points that need to be considered when contemplating the use of instrumental feedback devices. These include (1) physical and physiological factors (palatal tolerance for the instrumentation, attentional ability, etc.), (2) psychological factors (intellectual capabilities, learning difficulties, motivation, etc.), (3) personal factors (education, familial expectations, etc.), and (4) metalinguistic awareness of speech as combinations of individual sounds.

Use of instrumentally generated feedback as a remedial technique is relatively new within the practice of speech-language pathology. The availability of the instruments and the cost and training necessary to use them is somewhat limiting at this time. However, clinicians need to be aware of this aspect of the field which is growing into greater and greater prominence. The efficacious use of such instrumentation to assist in the modification of speech sound disorders, including DAS, needs to be objectively assessed. Once established, they may provide objective demonstrations of the efficacy of treatment.

Vowel and Dipthong Remediation Techniques

A characteristic of children with DAS that typifies the disorder is the presence of vowel and dipthong misarticulations. As described and discussed in Chapter 2, vowel errors are often clinically reported and transcribed in an inventory of errors produced by this population of children. Once vowel errors are identified, remedial planning should begin. However, Pollock (personal communication, 1992) shares a number of problems with the current state of the art regarding remediation of vowel errors. Clinical experience would indicate that some children occasionally self-correct vowel errors, but not many children with DAS have this experience. Many decisions must be made regarding vowels within a treatment program, such as whether vowel or consonant errors should be initially addressed or whether they should be targeted simultaneously. Other issues include the order in which vowel errors should be targeted in remediation and whether the ordering of the targeted consonant and vowel errors should be the same for the child with DAS as would be the practice with a child who does not present DAS but who does exhibit vowel errors. Much has yet to be learned about strategies and techniques for vowel remediation.

Pollock (personal communication, 1992) suggests that we assess vowels for stimulability as we do consonants. Modeling, in the form of auditory cues supplied by the clinician, should be used. If the vowel is stimulable, there is some degree of optimism that the vowel can be modified through such modeling. Lack of stimulability suggests that modification of the error will require more highly specialized techniques. The catch is that, to date, very little of our professional knowledge and literature has addressed vowel misarticulations. Thus, the clinician is left with few resources upon which to draw in developing a remedial program. Work with vowels is perhaps more difficult than work with consonants because the phonemes are produced by shaping the oral cavity. Oral landmarks, articulatory targets, and lingual movements are not used in the same way they are used with intervention of consonantal errors. Consequently, vowel therapy is elusive, frustrating, and often appears to be avoided.

The literature in the area of vowel elicitation is admittedly small. Bosley (1981) presents information regarding vowel production characteristics and retraining techniques for so-called functional articulatory defects which the clinician may find helpful. However, much of the information on vowel remediation was developed from habilitation/education of individuals with specific types of communication disorders such as hearing impairments. Little empirical work has been conducted on the few techniques that are available. Most vowel elicitation techniques are used in remediation sequences similar to those used in treating consonant errors. Remediation of vowels is an area of clinical work that needs to be developed because of the impact of vowel production on intelligibility. Research on refinement of clinical strategies will be a contribution to the treatment of a variety of communication disorders. We present the following reported techniques for the sake of completeness. They may be helpful to individual clinicians and their clients with DAS and spur interest in treatment of this aspect of speech sound disorders.

Northampton (Yale) Vowel Chart

According to Davis and Hardick (1981), the Northampton, or Yale, charts were developed at the Clarke School for the Deaf in 1885 and were revised in 1925. Like many of the vowel habilitation techniques, the Northampton charts use visual, written (printed) cues to facilitate speech production. These charts use orthographic symbols consisting of letters of the English alphabet that occur in the students' printed curricular materials. Thus, the student does not need to learn any special symbols. Charts were developed for both consonants and vowels.

The Northampton vowel chart organizes vowels into three groups— back round vowels, front vowels, and diphthongs—and is used as an articulation/pronunciation guide. The symbols are presented along with an auditory presentation of the targeted vowel phoneme. The inclusion of the symbols would be possible at any level of speech task complexity.

Davis and Hardick (1981) describe this system as complex, necessitated by the variety of pronunciation rules used in American English. Davis and Hardick also note that the symbols "do not provide a completely accurate representation of English, but they constitute a helpful pronunciation guide that is widely used with hearing-impaired children" (p. 269). No efficacy studies are reported by Davis and Hardick using hearing impaired, deaf, or normal hearing populations.

The Northampton charts have limitations. However, the system may offer a visual cuing system, and could be incorporated into a remedial program that is using another technique for consonant remediation. We have not used the system and we are not advocating its adoption by clinicians. However, it may be an avenue to explore.

Alcorn Symbols

The Alcorn symbols were developed by Streng in 1955. The symbols purport to visually represent the mouth shapes assumed during production of vowels and diphthongs. According to Davis and Hardick (1981), the purpose of the symbols is to help the child associate the written symbol and the oral movement.

The symbols can be used in a variety of ways and with a variety of ages. The system would need to be taught systematically, beginning with selected symbols and vowels and carefully expanded in number as success warrants. Task complexity also needs to be controlled, starting with isolated vowels and gradually increasing the difficulty of the speech task. Davis and Hardick (1981) state that the symbols are used with very young children by drawing faces with the symbols on paper plates, to be used as flashcards or as cues/reminders in speech activities. The symbols can also be combined with letters so that older children with some reading skills could associate the sequence of phonemes involved in an entire production.

Davis and Hardick (1981) report no research using this technique with children with hearing impairment, the population for which it was developed. Clinically, we have used the technique with one school-aged client with multiple disabilities, who presented a suspected mixed dysarthria and DAS. Unfortunately, use of the technique was not systematically studied so our comments are retrospective. We initially taught the symbols slowly and systematically in CV and CVC syllables. The symbols were all drawn onto pictured or written stimulus cards. In the case of written stimulus words, we first used only the symbol not the letter. Later we drew the symbol above the written vowel grapheme, slowly fading their inclusion the client's performance seemed to indicate less and less need for the visual cue. Finally visual cues were eliminated completely. Correct vowel phonemes were maintained in all but lengthy multisyllabic words.

Adapted Cuing Technique (ACT), Moto-kinesthetic, and Speech Facilitation

Please refer to descriptions contained in the earlier sections of this chapter.

Instrumental Feedback

Instrumentation, discussed in an earlier section of this chapter, could contribute to vowel remediation. Povel and Wansink (1986) described use of such instrumental feedback with eight deaf children between 8 and 14 years of age. They reported that the children found the visual feedback of the "vowel corrector" to be motivating and reinforcing. The system allowed for intensity differences that the deaf children were able to use for successful correction. Problems arose in training spectrally similar vowels because of the overlap between vowels.

Fletcher and Hasegawa (1983) reported on a visual articulatory modeling and feedback program developed for a 3½-year-old deaf child. The training program targeted the vowels /i/ and /a/, using instrumentally generated displays of both tongue position and movements, with the goal of developing high-low vowel contrasts in spoken words. Several consonants were targeted as well. An orometric system was developed to assess the child's speech production patterns and included the collection of palatometric, gnathometric, and glossometric measures. Results of the study suggested that visual articulatory displays were helpful to the child when developing articulatory actions and timing control.

These studies suggest that instrumental approaches have promise in the habilitation of vowel errors. Speech-language pathologists should not fear being replaced by a computer but should learn to use it to assist them in their work when financial resources allow for the acquisition of such technology.

Miscellaneous

Vowel errors are often difficult to modify and may require imagination and creativity on the part of the clinician. The following are several additional thoughts using visual and auditory cues that clinicians may find helpful in pursuing vowel modification.

Visual cues may be provided by use of dictionary diacritical marks. These would be similar in use in remediation to other types of visual cues such as the Alcorn symbols but are also tied closely to academic instruction. The symbols are letters, or graphemes, with which the child may feel comfortable. It is suggested that the clinician consult and coordinate with the child's educational team, however, before initiating such remedial instruction so that information gained in therapy is consistent with the instructional dictionary being used in the child's classroom or school.

We have hypothesized that color coding vowels may be another visual cue that could be helpful to the child with DAS who has unimpaired color perception. Color coding could be used in a variety of ways and would probably be more helpful in the sequencing of vowels with other phonemes rather than in the actual elicitation of the phoneme itself. Further, color systems may help the child anticipate when a vowel sound is to appear in the sequence of visually presented stimuli and how the vowel is to be sequenced with other phonemes. There are a number of ways in which the colors could help: a different color could be used for each vowel, a single color could indicate the presence of any specific vowel, or a color family could represent groups of vowels such as high-front vowels or low-back vowels.

The auditory channel may be used in many ways to evoke correct vowel productions. One strategy involves use of auditory bombardment in which the clinician provides multiple models of a selected phoneme, in this case a vowel, and produces many words that contain the targeted sound. This may help the child focus on the targeted phoneme and gain salient information about its production. A second strategy, reported by Pollock (personal correspondence, 1992), is that "choral" responses may help evoke correct production. These responses are made by the child, who produces the stimulus simultaneously with the clinician. Perhaps this allows the child to monitor, on-line, their production attempts and therefore to make whatever minute changes are needed in order to match the vowel produced by the clinician. A third strategy includes work with minimal pairs to also facilitate the development of the correct vowel use in words. The contrasts also help the child appreciate the importance of the correct vowel for intelligibility and making their needs known.

CHAPTER 9

Specific Issues Associated with the Communication Remediation of Children with DAS

C hildren with DAS offer the speech-language professional many challenges. Because children with DAS often present multiple communication problems, the clinician with such a child on his/her caseload is faced with numerous questions on how to best serve the child and the child's total needs. This chapter will address several management issues that occur within the context of DAS intervention.

Augmentative and Alternative Communication (AAC)

Augmentative and Alternative Communication (AAC) possibilities are a relevant consideration in the practice of speech-language pathology and audiology. McCormick and Shane (1990) describe the slow development of this area during the 1960s and early 1970s, possibly due to concerns that use of augmentative communication systems would interfere with the natural acquisition of speech. Fortunately, attitudes have changed and technology has advanced. Concerns for hearing clients whose communication abilities are limited, including some children with DAS, now seem to focus on helping them achieve functional communication in any way.

We use the term "alternative" communication to describe systems developed for those individuals who are unable, or are unlikely, to develop oral communication skills. "Augmentative" communication options are ones that do not replace speech, as is the case with alternative communication systems, but are options that can augment, enhance, or support the person's verbal communication attempts. Some augmentative and alternative communication options are aided, while others are unaided. Unaided options do not require any devices or equipment external to the body and include manual communication systems, gestures, etc. Aided options require some type of equipment external to the body such as paper and pencil, communication boards, communication books, etc.

Sign/Total Communication

One of the most frequently asked questions we receive from clinicians dealing with clients presenting severe DAS is: "Should I teach the child sign language?" This topic is also one of parental concern. The question often comes from the frustration of little, if any, appreciable progress being made when remedial goals target oral speech production. The clinician recognizes the need to help the child communicate in some manner. A reasonable consideration would be to use an unaided augmentative communication system such as sign language. Yet there is, perhaps, the fear that if allowed an easy way out of communicating, the child will rely on it and not strive to acquire speech skills.

It has been our clinical experience, from observation as well as by parental report, that children with DAS frequently develop some system of gestures on their own during preschool years, which allows them to communicate, even though minimally. Hall, Hardy, and LaVelle (1990) reported on a client and noted that her communication strategy included grunting, pointing, and a form of sign language that an older brother had taught her. The use of spontaneously developed gestures by children with DAS has been documented by others in the literature as well (Culp, 1989; Ferry, Hall, & Hicks, 1975; Harlan, 1984; McLaughlin & Kriegsmann, 1980).

Given that some type of gesturing is likely to be present during communication attempts, it seems logical to capitalize upon this and use it to help the child gain more control over the world. This would seem to be particularly important for those children with severe DAS. Jaffe (1984) defines *total communication* as a combination of speech with all modes of communication, particularly manual communication. She suggests that total communication be introduced to clients with DAS as an initial remedial strategy, and that it not be reserved for use only as a "last resort." Presumably, this suggestion would be applied to children who had not developed their own idiosyncratic gestures, as well as those who had. Jaffe's rationales for the suggestion that total communication be the first remedial approach to use with children exhibiting DAS were: (1) the child had not experienced failure with the gesture system as he or she had with speech attempts; (2) the visual channel is used, which Jaffe purported to be stronger than the auditory channel; (3) the child receives visual feedback via watching their own hands during gestures; (4) fine motor competence is not required for gestures as it is for speech; (5) the clinician can assist the client by molding and shaping the hands, which is not possible in the mouth in order to assist oral communication; (6) the signs can be statically maintained, allowing for extended duration, while speech is dynamic and changing; (7) the iconicity of sign language may facilitate language development; and (8) meaningful gross motor movements inherent in signs may be associated by the child with units of speech. Based on these rationales, Jaffe proposed a therapy program for children with moderate, as well as severe DAS, which extensively used total communication involving manual sign language and the manual alphabet. Early in the remedial program, sign language was suggested as the primary communication system with later use of signs and finger spelling to augment verbal communication. Jaffe suggests that signs may help the child recall and correctly produce speech sound patterns, as well as produce correct syntactical sequences. Jaffe also suggests that to be most effective, a total communication program needs to "emphasize meaning, spontaneous communication and consequences of communicative acts, not imitation, repetition and drill" (p. 125).

Ferry, Hall, and Hicks (1975) also advocated that total communication therapy was the intervention technique of choice, and that it should be initiated at the earliest possible age. They suggest that when *Developmental Verbal Dyspraxia* (DVD) is suspected, a trial period of intensive (defined as "daily") speech therapy be conducted with an "experienced" clinician for no longer than 6 months. If improvement is not achieved in that time period, alternative forms of therapy, which we assume to include manual communication systems, should be considered. Recall that Ferry, Hall, and Hicks also suggested that intelligible speech was unlikely to develop if this had not occurred by 6 years of age. This again underscores the importance of the development of manual communication skills by children with DVD in their philosophy of treating the disorder.

Air, Wood, and Neils (1989) present a slightly different perspective of the place of sign language in the treatment of children with DAS. They state that sign language can be used to augment communication if the child's language comprehension and cognitive abilities are better than their verbal skills. They suggest using this form of communication until verbal abilities "further develop." They advocate that the teaching of signs "should not preclude" remedial work in the areas of improved articulation or oral-motor skills.

The literature contains two case reports that deal with the use of sign language with clients exhibiting DAS. Harlan (1984) reports a case study that details the procedures she successfully used in a remedial program with concurrent nonspeech and oral treatment procedures. Culp (1989) wrote about a child who demonstrated a severe developmental speech apraxia, and who used signs and a picture communication book to help her communicate. The subject and her mother participated in an augmentative communication workshop where augumentative methods were assessed and an intervention program targeting improving functional and rewarding interactions between children using AAC (Alternative and Augmentative Communication) and their communication partners. Initial evaluation indicated that the child had frequent communication breakdowns, and that her signs lacked clarity. Pretests also revealed that she did not use her communication book to assist when communication failures occurred. Culp reported several types of measures that were taken pre-intervention and 2 months later. These results included that at the time of the posttest, the mother had reduced domination of the communicative interactions (from 75% to 63%). Also at posttest, using sign, the child more frequently offered information but less frequently answered yes/no or other types of questions; the child also improved in her ability to establish a topic of conversation. It was noted that her preference for the use of sign and gestures continued after the completion of the intervention phase of the study, this despite several modifications to enhance the utility and convenience of the communication book.

A compelling reason for including sign language within remedial programming is the child's newfound ability to communicatively interact in some way, which is denied when only verbal communication is encouraged or allowed. Rapin and Allen (1981) comment that "very severely affected children may be frustrated by their inability to communicate effectively and may exhibit a variety of behavior disorders. . . . Teaching the children sign language is . . . very helpful . . . because the signs provide the child with a channel to make known his desires" (p. 33). This seeming benefit has been reported by several authors who have noted the spontaneous modification of behavioral problems exhibited by children with DAS after the initiation of some type of manual communication. In a case study by McLaughlin and Kriegsmann (1980), the rapid learning and use of a core vocabulary of signs was reported so that the child could express his immediate needs. Concurrent with this improvement in communication, the disappearance of his extremely difficult behavior was noted. Ferry, Hall, and Hicks (1975) made a similar behavioral observation.

An often stated reservation expressed by referring clinicians and parents before the initiation of manual communication instruction is concern that once a child with DAS has been taught and uses a manual form of communication, he or she will use it solely to the detriment of the learning or acquisition of oral communication skills. Our experience, and that of others in the literature (Blackstone, 1989; Ferry, Hall, & Hicks, 1975; Harlan, 1984; McLaughlin & Kriegsmann, 1980) has found this *not* to be the case. As a child's oral proficiency improves, the need for and use of sign language seems to spontaneously fade until oral productions alone convey their messages. The signs may be used initially to help the child in some way to orally produce the target and to ensure the receiving of the message by the intended audience. As proficiency improves, these needs are no longer present so the signing system is eliminated in favor of attempts at the more efficient oral productions.

The role of the parent(s), caregiver, and other significant adults in implementing a treatment program involving a manual communication system is an important one. An initial hurdle may be one of attitude. One set of parents with whom we worked refused to consider this option for their son with severe developmental apraxia of speech because they thought his overt use of signs would label him as "handicapped" to those around him. In contrast, another set of legal guardians were so strongly in favor of this approach with their grandson exhibiting severe apraxia that they petitioned their school district for the hiring of a signing aide to be in his classroom and interpret his signing for the nonsigning teacher and classmates. Fortunately for the child, this accommodation was granted by the school system and became an integral part of his educational program and growth.

In order to be effective, everyone in a child's environment should ideally learn the system being taught to the child. This is a large time commitment, a commitment which some teachers may not feel they can make in order to work with a particular child in their classroom for only a single academic year. As we have stated before, clinicians working with children presenting DAS are often put in the role of becoming their advocates on a number of issues. Likewise, primary caregivers must also make the commitment to learn the sign system being taught to their child. By becoming more fluent signers themselves, the parents can facilitate their child's progress in remediation since the time they spend with the child far exceeds the time the clinician spends with the child, thus providing additional practice with the skill. As the parents become proficient readers of their child's sign they facilitate and reinforce communication with the child.

There are several sign or manual communication, systems presently in use, each with strengths and weaknesses. These factors need to be considered when selecting which particular manual system might best suit a child's needs or communication level. McCormick and Shane (1990) contrast the advantages and disadvantages of several systems, including Signed English, American Sign Language (ASL), fingerspelling, simultaneous (total) communication, and pantomime and natural gesture.

It is our opinion that the use of sign or other manual communication systems has a place within the overall remedial programming for children with DAS. The specific issues of which system to use, when to initiate this aspect of service, whether to use sign solely or to supplement oral goals, how the system will serve the child's growth in communication skills, etc., are ones that the clinician will need to address on an individual basis for each client in consultation with the parents and others on the child's team. Certainly the idiosyncratic gestures that children often develop on their own can be regularized into an established system of manual communication, further extending the group of individuals who know the signs and can thus communicate with the child. This, in turn, gives the child power and control over even minimal aspects of the world.

We also think that there is another positive gain that can evolve from the use of manual communication as a component of a remedial program for a child with DAS. Signing requires movements that are sequential in nature; speech requires the same. Thus, signing may help a child acquire a sense of sequential movements with some part of the body, which later may be successfully transferred to movements of the articulators for speech purposes. Clinical observations indicate that the use of sign does not impede oral communication development and may actually facilitate it. As speech skills improve, the use of signs reduces and may eventually drop out of the child's system of communication.

A caution: Recall that in earlier parts of the text we reported that children with DAS may also exhibit other forms of apraxia. The possible presence, and degree, of limb apraxia must be determined before a decision is made to include manual systems into remediation. In some cases limb apraxia may negate this as a viable option. In other cases the clinician, and other adults involved with the child, may need to make accommodations in the accuracy with which the signs are made by the child. Further, with these children, perhaps other types of alternative or augmentative communication devices or systems should be considered.

Aided Communication Techniques

Authors recognize the potential need for the use of aided alternative communication devices with some children exhibiting severe DAS (Ferry, Hall, & Hicks, 1975; Aram and Nation, 1982; Haynes, 1985; Blackstone, 1989; Culp, 1989). Specifically suggested are use of Bliss and Rebus symbols, language boards, special typewriters, electronic communication devices, and communication books. The practicing clinician may consider alternative devices to enhance verbal attempts or as the primary communication technique for a child with DAS when it appears that the prognosis for achieving functional verbal skills is not favorable.

There are numerous considerations that need to be taken into account when attempting to match the child with DAS with an alternative communication device. One is that the child with DAS is typically an ambulatory individual. Thus, the size and sturdiness of the unit must be taken into account. Small size may enhance portability for the child and therefore increase the probability of the devices' use when the child encounters communication breakdowns. However a small size may inherently limit the number of entries the device can contain which may be used by the child.

Culp (1989) identifies a second problem, which is how to appropriately select a functional vocabulary for the device. She points out that because children with DAS have motoric independence, they typically have experiences in a wide variety of environments and with a wide variety of people. Culp notes that these factors "require the availability of extensive and unpredictable vocabulary" (p. 32). Certainly, close contact with all significant people in a child's life is a necessity in order to determine the most salient vocabulary items for that child. The clinician must also recognize the need for frequent modifications and upgrades of vocabulary. We suggest that clinicians consider developing multiple vocabulary displays that reflect different facets of a child's life if these provide more flexibility for the child.

A third factor is the personal preferences of the child as to the type of device which best suits them. The communication book approach was apparently not successfully used with Culp's client; this same type of device was immediately endorsed and eagerly used by a client of ours. Thus, exposure to, and experience with, a number of possible devices is important for each child with DAS for whom alternative devices are being considered. A device that seems most suitable to the clinician (and parent) will not be helpful if the child does not also think that it is the most suitable.

Work with alternative communication devices is becoming a highly specialized area of professional expertise, with many professions having input into the development of this area. Current and future advances result in rapid changes in the technology of the devices. We suggest that a clinician who is seeing the need to suggest alternative devices for a child with DAS seek out individuals working in this highly specific area. For background information in the area, the reader is referred to Silverman, 1980; Blackstone, 1989; and McCormick and Shane, 1990.

Cognitive/Conceptual/Linguistic/Phonological Remedial Approaches

Much of the current assessment and treatment of speech sound disorders is completed via use of techniques addressing distinctive features, minimal pairs, contrasts, and phonological processes. Theoretically, this viewpoint holds that the errors are based on difficulties in learning the rules inherent in the phonologic aspect of language. The child discovers, then acquires, rule-governed knowledge about her/his language, including the speech sound system. The goals of remediation are to help the child modify the rule system so that it nears that of the adult standard, measured by improved intelligibility thus facilitating communication in general. The problem is described as cognitively-, conceptually-, linguistically-, or phonologically-based.

Several references suggest that phonological remediation be used with children exhibiting DAS. Hodson (1989) commented that a phonological processes approach that uses cycles was adaptable enough to be appropriate for children with the diagnosis of *developmental dyspraxia.* Hodson and Paden (1991) reported a remedial history of a child with an early diagnosis of dyspraxia, with positive efficacy reported anecdotally.

Intervention philosophies and programs are generated from the theoretical beliefs one holds about a disorder. Our orientation to the speech sound disorders presented by children with DAS is not language-based. It is based on a belief that the disorder is one of motor control (Hall, 1992; Robin, 1992). Therefore, we believe that the linguistically-based treatment philosophies are inadequate for children with DAS.

The literature supports this point of view with a number of statements that the phonological therapy approaches would not be appropriate for children with DAS. Stoel-Gammon and Dunn (1985) noted that "a basic level of motor ability is an essential prerequisite for success with conceptual treatment tasks" (p. 178). Creaghead (1989) noted that children exhibiting a number of selected diagnoses, including DAS, would not be appropriate candidates for linguistically-based approaches because "production rather than rule-learning may be the primary difficulty" (p. 195). Pannbacker (1988) notes "Developmental apraxia of speech is extremely resistant to . . . rule-based phonology approaches" (p. 364). Weiss, Gordon, and Lillywhite (1987) commented that the phonologic processes approach was "not (recommended) for phonetic deviances" (p. 220). Bernthal and Bankson (1988) include in their remedial guidelines for cognitive-linguistic approaches the statement that these approaches should not be used on speech sound errors that are motor-based.

Because of our motor-control orientation, we find it difficult to reconcile how phonological remediation, which is largely based on receptive input to the child, can facilitate improved prowess in the actual motor movements needed to produce speech sounds. Cognitive (re)organization of the language's system of phonemes would not seem to be consistent with our perceptions of the speech sound deficits exhibited by a child with DAS. At a cognitive level, many of the clients presenting DAS with whom we work seem to "know" what the targeted phoneme "sounds" like, as evidenced by their abilities to correctly evaluate the adequacy of their own productions. Rather, the problem seems to involve correctly executing the necessary articulatory movements, which result in the correct production of the speech sound. Further, we have reservations about the application of some linguistically-based programs because, when strictly executed, the programs do not seem to give sufficient time or practice opportunities for the child with DAS to master the articulatory gestures necessary for correct phoneme production and sequencing. We also have reservations that, for a child with DAS, too many phonemes may be targeted simultaneously, and the targeted phonemes may be rotated too rapidly so that production mastery is not achieved. Because of our orientation, we do not embrace remedial programming using phonological philosophies.

However, two of the techniques described for use in linguistically-based remediation might be used for individual children with DAS and could be appropriate to a motor-programming context. We stress that the techniques are used to enhance some aspect of motor-programming proficiency, not to help them acquire the rules of the phonological aspects of their language system.

With some children with DAS, auditory bombardment may help them focus on the phoneme being introduced to them. The focus may be a vowel or a consonant which seems to be particularly resistant to correct production. However, it has been our experience that such bombardment is not necessary for the majority of phonemes targeted with clients exhibiting DAS. Our inclusion of auditory bombardment is not intended to increase error-awareness because we find that many children with DAS hear their own speech and are very aware of their errors. The intent is the provision of intensive listening opportunities focused on phonemes with which the children are having particular difficulty, also including any specific elicitation techniques that assist in the actual production of the targeted phoneme(s). We believe, as Greene (1967) noted, "The dyspraxic . . . child needs to be taught how to articulate, and listening training *alone* is not enough" (p. 143).

A second activity that may be helpful in remediation with the client presenting DAS, although cited for use with language-based disorders, is incorporation of minimal pairs or similar contrasts, where effective communication is required for task success. Such activities may provide a child much helpful and communicatively salient practice when he or she is dealing with a goal of consistent and accurate production of contrasting phonemes. For instance, the minimal pairs approach may be very appropriate for a child who needs to develop the accurate and consistently correct voicing contrasts of cognate phonemes. Using such minimal contrasts as "pill" versus "bill" versus "ill" and "cap" versus "cab" might be useful to help a child learn to produce correct voicing of stops. Although the pool of possible real-word stimuli may be small because of the need for careful control over word structure, the corpus may be expanded by including nonsense words. Another way to manage the pool of potential contrastive words is suggested by Elbert and Gierut (1986), who suggest *near minimal pairs* (paired words sharing the same vowel adjacent to the targeted sound, although other phonemes in the words may differ). Marquardt and Sussman (1991) described the multiple remedial approaches used with the client in their case study. Contrasting minimal pairs had been used during three semesters of therapy with the child and they concluded that progress was made when the targeted pairs contained sounds with similar placement (we assume not manner or voicing) features. This information may be helpful to the clinician in evaluating the possible incorporation of this technique into a remedial program.

Working with Preschoolers Exhibiting DAS

During our conversations with practicing speech-language pathologists, we are frequently asked about how best to serve preschoolers with suspected DAS. We choose to use the words "suspected DAS" because it has been our experience that diagnostic certainty is often very difficult, although not impossible, with a child in the preschool age range. As with older children, we have found that we may be reasonably comfortable with a provisional diagnosis of DAS but observations over a longer period of time may confirm or negate that possible diagnosis with a preschool aged child. Nonetheless, it is also our belief that early identification of a communication disorder and provision of appropriate services is essential. To underscore the importance of services to the preschool child, eventual outcome may be related to the age at which appropriate services were initiated. Lohr (1978) stated that with her population of nonverbal clients with apraxia, "children who were younger when we began working with them progressed more rapidly" (p. 6). Our experience has been that the overall outcome has been best for those children with DAS who were identified as possibly exhibiting DAS and received services as very young children. Ferry, Hall, and Hicks (1975) shared their opinion that if intelligible speech had not developed by 6 years of age with a child exhibiting developmental verbal dyspraxia, "it was unlikely to develop". Although this opinion is not universally shared, it does emphasize the importance of services for the preschooler with DAS.

The development of a diagnosis may be the result of a period of diagnostic therapy, where numerous hypotheses about the child's speech sound disorder may be tested. For instance, games involving the imitation of articulator movements should be attempted. This affords the opportunity to compare and contrast the imitated movements with spontaneous movements and postures the child makes during the sessions. This information may be helpful in determining how well the child and his/her mechanism functions in a volitional context. Activities could also be adapted to gain insights into the mechanism's abilities to complete both speech and nonspeech movements upon command. Performance of these types of activities may help the clinician determine whether a child exhibits an adequate structural mechanism, one which has some suspected degree of motor involvement or motor-control involvement such as dysarthria, apraxia, or both.

The verbalizations of the preschoolers also need to be observed, transcribed, and analyzed. The size of the phonemic repertoire and its consistent use in communicative attempts needs to be noted. If the child is not yet verbal, the vocalizations and nonspeech sounds the child produces needs to be observed, described, and analyzed. The variety of vocal sounds, use of pitch contours, and consistency of use in communication attempts should be noted.

Because children with DAS frequently have co-occurring and associated problems (see Chapters 4, 5, and 6), careful observations of the preschool child, in toto, is necessary. This includes such essentials as receptive and expressive language skills, fine and gross motor skills, general learning style, etc.

A preschool child with a severe or profound communication disorder can be a very intimidating client because there seem to be an overwhelming number of problems that demand attention. When such a child is suspected of exhibiting DAS the clinician has many decisions to make in establishing remedial goals.

With a child suspected of DAS who exhibits few verbal communication skills, the clinician may need to consider initiating a manual communication system. As discussed previously in this chapter, manual communication may provide a way for a child to express himself or herself. The strategy may also assist the child in gaining practice in producing sequential motor movements. Such practice may positively influence the organization of the motor movements involved in speech production.

Many clinicians report that they use phonological processes approaches with their preschool clients who exhibit some verbalization and vocalization. With a preschool population, a processes program of intervention could provide helpful information about the child's abilities to acquire speech production skills. If the child makes changes, as seen in the emergence of phonemes and increased speech intelligibility, the clinician may conclude that the child's problems are phonological in nature and may choose to continue this treatment approach. However, if the child does not exhibit phoneme emergence and is observed to exhibit behaviors used to describe DAS, we suggest a change in therapy philosophy to more directly deal with sound production skills via motor-programming remediation approaches.

Speech production goals with the preschool child exhibiting DAS must be developed to address the unique problems of the individual child. We suggest adaptations of motor-programming remediation principles when working with preschoolers with DAS. Some children may need to work on gross motor imitative skills as a precursor to eventual imitation of the articulator movements involved in speech sound production. Other children may need to learn vocal/verbal imitation skills through production of "noises" such as animal sounds, vehicular sounds, etc. If a child produces even one phoneme, imitatively or spontaneously, the clinician should demand consistent production of it, following the general motor-programming hierarchy discussed earlier in Chapter 7. Normal developmental sequence and visibility of phonemes should be considered when setting goals. Accommodations for the preschooler must include developing stimuli relevant to the age and interests of the child, modifying length of sessions, developing reinforcers that are age-appropriate, etc. As well, other aspects of the child's total communication problems may need to be addressed in goal setting.

The speech-language clinician may need to serve as an early advocate for additional services that the young child with DAS may need, such as early childhood educational programming and involvement of physical therapists or occupational therapists. The speech-language clinician then works as a team member within the total programming for the child.

Preschoolers with suspected DAS are a challenging population for the speech-language professional. Good observational skills are needed, as well as the ability to be flexible and creative in modifying goals and activities to best help the individual child.

CHAPTER 10

The Future Is Yours

The body of available literature dealing with the topic of developmental apraxia of speech (DAS) has numerous citations generated from diverse sources and professions. Perhaps it is important to reflect on the history of this literature to better understand the study of the disorder, which, in turn, may help us understand where we are today and what paths might be explored in the future.

While the initial description of the disorder (Hadden, 1891) is now over 100 years old, much of the literature, especially that originating in the United States, is relatively new. Prior to 1970, occasional reference was made to this population of children, particularly in subsections of textbooks. However, the 1970s saw a distinct and active interest in this clinical area with the information being conveyed in the more easily accessible and widely distributed speech-language pathology professional journals. Much of this literature consisted of anecdotal reports, case studies, and several data-based empirical studies.

In 1981, Guyette and Diedrich published a book chapter titled ''A Critical Review of Developmental Apraxia of Speech.'' They noted numerous problems with the body of research and were particularly critical of research designs and contradictory or inconclusive results. Based on their interpretation of the literature, Guyette and Diedrich concluded that ''the diagnosis 'developmental apraxia of speech' is neither appropriate nor useful'' (p. 44). While helpful in pointing out problems within the literature, perhaps Guyette and Diedrich's chapter was a disservice since its effect may have been to hinder further growth in the knowledge base. The ''does exist'' versus ''does not exist'' arguments about the disorder came more sharply into focus. Meanwhile, many clinicians continued to find the concept of DAS helpful in their practice of speech-language pathology, despite differences of opinion regarding the theoretical underpinnings and the degree of stringency in the research efforts devoted to the topic. More recently there appears, once again, to be an acceleration in the research and clinical efforts to explore the concept and/or disorder of DAS, which, hopefully, is being conducted with carefully considered research designs.

We must also be sensitive to the evolutionary process that is involved in gaining an understanding of clinical entities such as DAS. Deputy (1984) stated that the scientific method begins with documented observations which advances to careful descriptions and then advances to explanations and predictions. The DAS literature now contains frequent reports of observations and must advance to the level of carefully documenting those observations and objectively collecting descriptive information. The profession awaits explanations that permit prediction.

There are several methods by which observations and descriptions can be made. Love (1992) notes several such methods. One is *equated groups,* used to determine if two or more groups differ on a given parameter(s). This research design is commonly used in behavioral research and was initially applied to the study of DAS by Yoss and Darley (1974a). However, Love expresses concerns about equated group research because of problems in defining DAS subject selection criterion across studies as well as the absence of non-DAS controls in some studies. He suggests that the case study approach provides evidence for the validity of developmental apraxia, as well as "to establish the nature of disorder . . . to test the efficacy of therapeutic techniques" (p. 105). He further notes that it is an approach used in the health sciences "to provide descriptions of unusual cases and to offer new information about poorly understood disorders" (p. 105). A third methodology that may hold promise in the study of DAS is that of single subject design (McReynolds & Kearns, 1983). The multiple baseline design should be particularly useful in assessing which type of treatment best works with children exhibiting DAS. It is imperative that the efficacy of our clinical efforts be tested.

We suggest that the following are examples of the numerous directions that future research efforts in the study of DAS might explore. We caution that our suggestions are not meant to imply that these are the only directions in which there might be productive work.

Needs We Continue to Identify

1. The nature and characteristics of the disorder need to be better defined. In the future we may be able to define consistent characteristics of the disorder. A cluster of symptoms may be agreed upon as constituting the disorder. The differences, if any, between children with DAS and children who exhibit functional/developmental/ phonological speech sound disorders may be defined. The contribution of motor programming to the nature of DAS may be better appreciated. The changes, over time,

in the characteristics of DAS need to be described, as does the impact of different treatment programs. Larger numbers of children with suspected DAS should be carefully studied in a number of communication areas, as well as a number of related areas such as language skills, academic skills, and social skills. Along these lines it is necessary to determine if children with DAS can be identified from a larger group of children with speech sound disorders on the basis of the symptoms used to define DAS.

2. The theoretical constructs that may explain DAS need to be empirically explored with adults and children and with normal and disordered communication skills. Methodologically sound studies would enhance this level of explanation, as would further documentation of models of normal and disordered motor control.

3. Etiological factors need to be explored and determined. Neurological etiologies have been suspected by a number of professionals to be the bases for DAS. The presence or absence of neurological factors needs to be documented, both for "soft" as well as "hard" neurological signs. Other neurological areas might also be explored to better describe brain function (e.g., blood flow, metabolic and chemical studies). Rapid advances in this area of medicine make this a potentially exciting area of future exploration.

4. The potential relationship between oral, nonverbal apraxias, and DAS needs to be explored using paradigms that accurately assess movement control during speech and nonspeech activities.

5. The possible role of DAS in the definition of various medically diagnosed syndromes and metabolic disorders has been alluded to in the literature. This is an area of emerging importance, requiring careful documentation and description.

6. Standardized assessment procedures and instruments need to be developed that will assist in the diagnosis of the disorder. This might be done with either (or both) existing and new protocols. Research in this area would need to be done with care in the development of the psychometric characteristics of the instrument (McCauley & Swisher, 1984a; McCauley and Swisher, 1984b; Salvia &

Ysseldyke, 1991). Of particular interest would be the need to define, very carefully, the normal and disordered populations with which the procedures would be standardized. This should include a careful definition of the criterion characteristics on which the subjects with DAS were selected. Moreover, the accuracy of our diagnostic tools, and our own diagnostic skills, needs to be assessed. One such method might be to apply signal detection theory to the diagnostic setting (Swets & Pickett, 1982). For instance, the accuracy of aphasia diagnosis has been evaluated using signal detection measures (Robin & McNeil, 1992).

7. The factors which predict the occurrence of DAS in any particular child need to be identified, as do the possible familial trends, genetic predispositions, and factors in the early developmental history of the child.

8. The prevalence and incidence of DAS need to be documented.

9. If gender is a factor in the expression of the disorder, the ratio of boys to girls with the disorder needs to be identified. The severity of the problems by gender also needs to be described.

10. The total educational profiles of children with DAS needs to be systemically investigated. Professionals need to define the prevalence of problems in mathematics, reading, and spelling. These evaluations must take into account the child's growth through remediation of DAS, and growth in academic skills. This may identify the most helpful educational strategies in the learning processes of the child with DAS, as well as identify the strategies that are most helpful in reducing or minimizing the negative impact of the speech sound disorder on the educational instruction of the child.

11. The numerous treatment strategies purported to be of assistance to the child with DAS need to be systemically studied. Efficacy studies must be conducted to demonstrate any particular method's ability to yield positive change in the communication skills of a child exhibiting DAS. The most advantageous scheduling as to the intensity and timing in the delivery of services needs to be determined. Many of the present methods deal with modification of consonants. However, with a popula-

tion of children exhibiting DAS, remediation of vowels errors must also be addressed when remedial efficacy is studied. Other areas that need empirical exploration are alternative and assistive communication systems and devices. The systems that may facilitate or enhance communication for the child with DAS need to be identified. The hypothesis that the early use of manual communication systems with young children facilitates eventual verbal skills needs to be explored. The use of instrumental feedback within the remedial and diagnostic setting must be systematically investigated.

12. The outcome for children with DAS as they achieve adulthood must be described. The communication outcome is one of many quality-of-life issues that needs to be determined for this group of clients, which also includes educational history and vocational choice.

13. There is a critical need for the development of understandable informational materials about all aspects of DAS, written for the parents of children with the disorder. These same materials could also be useful to other lay persons such as educators who know and interact with children exhibiting the problem. Such materials would provide information that is badly needed to help make sense of a confusing disorder.

This chapter addresses but a few of the numerous issues that we hope will serve to focus questions that need to be asked in the study of DAS. The goals of this text are to attempt to compile and review the presently known literature and to share our experience with, and views of, the disorder. It is our belief that an active future awaits DAS, with further explorations and understandings about the disorder generating from these efforts. The future promises to be exciting if carefully controlled systematic investigation resulting in empirical evidence is accomplished. A commitment to continued interest and careful study is needed as we explore the elusive disorder known as Developmental Apraxia of Speech.

References

Adams, C. (1990). Syntactic comprehension in children with expressive language impairment. *British Journal of Disorders of Communication, 25,* 149–171.

Air, D. H., & Wood, A. S. (1985). Considerations for organic disorders. In P. W. Newman, N. A. Creaghead, & W. Secord (Eds.), *Assessment and remediation of articulatory and phonological disorders* (pp. 269–281). Columbus: Charles E. Merrill.

Air, D. H., Wood, A. S., & Neils, J. R. (1989). Considerations for organic disorders. In N. A. Creaghead, P. W. Newman, & W. A. Secord (Eds.), *Assessment and remediation of articulatory and phonological disorders,* 2nd ed., (pp. 265–301). Columbus: Merrill Publishing Company.

Albert, M., Sparks, R., & Helm, N. (1973). Melodic intonation therapy for aphasia. *Archives of Neurology, 29,* 130–131.

Aram, D. M. (1980). *Whatever happened to functional articulation disorders?* Paper presented at the annual meeting of the American Speech-Language-Hearing Association, Detroit.

Aram, D. M. (1982). *Developmental verbal apraxia: A disorder in search of definition.* Unpublished manuscript, Case Western Reserve University, Rainbow Babies' and Children's Hospital, Department of Pediatrics, Cleveland, Ohio.

Aram, D. M. (1984). Preface. In W. H. Perkins & J. L. Northern (Eds.), *Seminars in speech and language* (unnumbered pages). New York: Thieme-Stratton.

Aram, D. M., & Glasson, C. (1979). *Developmental apraxia of speech.* Paper presented at the annual meeting of the American Speech-Language-Hearing Association, Atlanta.

Aram, D. M., & Horwitz, S. J. (1981). *Sequential abilities and nonspeech practic abilities in developmental verbal apraxia.* Manuscript with portions presented at the annual meeting of the American Speech Hearing Association, Los Angeles.

Aram, D. M., & Nation, J. E. (1982). *Child language disorders* (pp. 144–249). St. Louis: C. V. Mosby.

Arthur, G. (1952). *The Arthur adaptation of the Leiter international performance scale.* Washington, DC: Psychological Service Center Press.

Aten, J. (1979). *Denver auditory phoneme sequencing test.* Houston: College Hill Press.

Aten, J., & Davis, J. (1968). Disturbances in the perception of auditory sequence in children with minimal cerebral dysfunction. *Journal of Speech and Hearing Research, 11,* 236–245.

Aten, J. L., Johns, D. F., & Darley, F. L. (1971). Auditory perception of sequenced words in apraxia of speech. *Journal of Speech and Hearing Research, 14,* 131–143.

Barlow, S. M., & Abbs, J. M. (1986). Fine force and position control of select oro-facial structures in upper motor neuron syndrome. *Experimental Neurology, 94,* 699–713.

Bashir, A. S., Grahamjones, F., & Bostwick, R. Y. (1984). A touch-cue method of therapy for developmental verbal apraxia. In W. H. Perkins & J.L. Northern (Eds.), *Seminars in speech and language* (pp. 127–137). New York: Thieme-Stratton.

Benson, D. F. (1979). *Aphasia, alexia, and agraphia* (Clinical Neurology and Neurosurgery Monographs, Vol. 1). New York: Churchill Livingstone.

Bernthal, J. E., & Bankson, N. W. (1988). *Articulation and phonological disorders* (2nd ed.). Englewood Cliffs, NJ: Prentice-Hall.

Betsworth, M. K., & Hall, P. K. (1989). *The presence of variability in developmental apraxia of speech.* Paper presented at the annual meeting of the American Speech-Language-Hearing Association, St. Louis.

Bilodeau, I. M. (1956). Accuracy of a simple positioning response with variation in the number of trials by which knowledge of results is delayed. *American Journal of Psychology, 69,* 434–437.

Bilodeau, I. M. (1966). Information feedback. In E. A. Bilodeau (Ed.), *Acquisition of skill* (pp. 255–296). New York: Academic Press.

Bilodeau, I. M. (1969). Information feedback. In E. A. Bilodeau (Ed.), *Principles of skill acquisition* (pp. 255–285). New York: Academic Press.

Blackstone, S. W. (1989). Those who walk: In search of better solutions. *Augmentative Commmunication News, 2,* 1–4.

Blakeley, R. W. (1980). *Screening test for developmental apraxia of speech.* Tigard, Oregon: C. C. Publications.

Blakeley, R. W. (1983). Treatment of developmental apraxia of speech. In W. H. Perkins (Ed.), *Dysarthria and apraxia* (pp. 25–33). New York: Thieme-Stratton.

Bosley, E. C. (1981). *Techniques for articulatory disorders.* Springfield, IL: Charles C. Thomas Publishers.

Bowman, S. N., Parsons, C. L., & Morris, D. A. (1984). Inconsistency of phonological errors in developmental verbal dyspraxic children as a factor of linguistic task and performance load. *Australian Journal of Human Communication Disorders, 12,* 109–119.

Bradley, D. P. (1989). A systematic multiple-phoneme approach. In N. A. Greaghead, P. W. Newman, & W. A. Secord (Eds.), *Assessment & remediation of articulatory and phonological disorders,* 2nd ed., (pp. 305–322). Columbus, OH: Merrill Publishing Co.

Bradley, D. P., & McCabe, R. B. (1971). A systematic multiple-sound approach to articulation remediation. Short course presented at the Annual Convention of the American Speech and Hearing Association, Chicago, IL.

Campbell, T., & Shriberg, L. D. (1982). Association among pragmatic functions, linguistic stress, and natural phonological processes in speech delayed children. *Journal of Speech and Hearing Research, 25,* 547–553.

Carrow, E. (1974). *Carrow elicited language inventory.* Allen, TX: DLM Teaching Resources.

Catts, H. (1989). Phonological processing deficits and reading disabilities. In A. Kamhi & H. Catts (Eds.), *Reading disabilities: A developmental language perspective* (pp. 101–132). San Diego, CA: College-Hill Press.

Chappell, G. E. (1973). Childhood verbal apraxia and its treatment. *Journal of Speech and Hearing Disorders, 38,* 362–368.

Chappell, G. E. (1984). Developmental verbal dyspraxia: The expectant pattern. *Australian Journal of Human Communication Disorders, 12,* 15–25.

Chumpelik, D. (1984). The PROMPT system of therapy: Theoretical framework and applications for developmental apraxia of speech. In W. H. Perkins & J. L. Northern (Eds.), *Seminars in speech and language* (pp. 139–155). New York: Thieme-Stratton.

Comeau, S., & Crary, M. A. (1982). *Developmental verbal dyspraxia: A morpho-phonemic analysis.* Miniseminar presented at the annual meeting of the American Speech-Language-Hearing Association, Toronto.

Compton, A. J. (1986). *Compton phonological assessment of children.* San Francisco: Carousel House.

Compton, A. J., & Hutton, J. S. (1978). *Compton-Hutton phonological assessment.* San Francisco: Carousel House.

Conrad, K. E., Cermak, S. A., & Drake, C. (1983). Differentiation of praxis among children. *American Journal of Occupational Therapy, 37,* 466–473.

Cooper, W. E., Eady, S. J., & Mueller, P. R. (1985). Acoustical aspects of contrastive stress in question-answer contexts. *Journal of the Acoustical Society of America, 77,* 2142–2156.

Cooper, W. E., & Sorensen, J. M. (1981). *Fundamental frequency in sentence production.* New York: Springer-Verlog.

Cornett, R. (1972). *Cued speech parent training and follow-up program.* Washington, DC: Bureau of Education for Handicapped, DHEW, 96.

Cosmides, L. (1983). Invariances in the acoustic expression of emotion during speech. *Journal of Experimental Psychology: Human Perception and Performance, 9,* 864–881.

Court, D., & Harris, M. (1965). Speech disorders in children: Part II. *British Medical Journal, 2,* 409–411.

Crary, M. A. (1981). *Phonological process analysis of developmental verbal dyspraxia: A descriptive study.* Paper presented at the annual meeting of the American Speech-Language-Hearing Association, Los Angeles.

Crary, M. A. (1982). *Developmental verbal dyspraxia: A phonological research perspective.* Miniseminar presented at the annual meeting of the American Speech-Language-Hearing Association, Toronto.

Crary, M. A. (1984a). A neurolinguistic perspective on developmental verbal dyspraxia. *Communicative Disorders, 9,* 33–47.

Crary, M. A. (1984b). Phonological characteristics of developmental verbal dyspraxia. In W. H. Perkins & J. L. Northern (Eds.), *Seminars in speech and language* (pp. 71–83). New York: Thieme-Stratton.

Crary, M. A., & Fokes, J. (1979). Phonological processes in apraxia of speech: A systematic simplification of articulatory performance. *Aphasia-Apraxia-Agnosia. 1*(4), 1–13.

Crary, M. A., Landess, S., & Towne, R. (1984). Phonolgical error patterns in developmental verbal dyspraxia. *Journal of Neuropsychology, 6,* 157–170.

Crary, M. A., & Towne, R. (1984). The asynergistic nature of developmental verbal dyspraxia. *Australian Journal of Human Communication Disorders, 12,* 27–37.

Creaghead, N. A. (1989). Linguistic approaches to treatment. In N. A. Creaghead, P. A. Newman, & W. A. Secord (Eds.), *Assessment and remediation of articulatory and phonological disorders*, 2nd ed. (pp. 193–215). Columbus, OH: Merrill Publishing Co.

Creaghead, N. A., Newman, P. W., & Secord, W. A. (Eds.) (1989). *Assessment and remediation of articulatory and phonological disorders* (2nd ed.). Columbus, OH: Merrill Publishing Company.

Cromer, R. F. (1978). The basis of childhood dysphasia: A linguistic approach. In M. A. Wyke (Ed.), *Developmental dysphasia* (pp. 85–134). New York: Academic Press.

Crystal, D. (1981). *Clinical linguistics.* New York: Springer-Verlag.

Culp, D. M. (1989). Developmental apraxia and augmentative or alternative communication—A case example. *AAC Augmentative and Alternative Communication.* (pp. 27–34) Baltimore: Williams & Wilkins.

Dabul, B. L. (1971). Lingual incoordination-language delay. *California Journal of Communication Disorders, 2,* 30–33.

Dabul, B. L., & Bollier, B. (1976). Therapeutic approaches to apraxia. *Journal of Speech and Hearing Disorders, 41,* 268–276.

Daly, D. A., Cantrell, R. P., Cantrell, M. L., & Aman, L. A. (1972). Structuring speech therapy contingencies with an oral apraxic child. *Journal of Speech and Hearing Disorders, 37,* 22–32.

Dare, M. T., & Gordon, N. (1970). Clumsy children: A disorder of perception and motor organization. *Developmental Medicine and Child Neurology, 12,* 178–185.

Darley, F. L. (1968). Apraxia of speech: 107 years of terminological confusion. Paper presented at the annual meeting of the American Speech and Hearing Association, Denver.

Darley, F. L., Aronson, A. E., & Brown, J. R. (1969). Clusters of deviant speech dimensions in the dysarthrias. *Journal of Speech and Hearing Research, 12,* 462–496.

Darley, F. L., Aronson, A. E., & Brown, J. R. (1975). *Motor speech disorders.* Philadelphia: W. B. Saunders.

Darley, F. L., & Spriestersbach, D. C. (Eds.). (1978). *Diagnostic methods in speech pathology* (2nd ed.). New York: Harper & Row.

Darwish, H., Pearce, P. S., Gaines, R., & Harasym, P. (1982). The speech programming deficit syndrome. *Annals of Neurology, 12,* 211.

Davis, B., Marquardt, T. P., & Sussman, H. M. (1985). *Developmental apraxia of speech: Case study.* Paper presented at the annual meeting of the American Speech-Language-Hearing Association, Washington, DC

Davis, J. M., & Hardick, E. J. (1981). *Rehabilitative audiology for children and adults.* New York: John Wiley & Sons.

Denays, R., Tondeur, M., Foulon, M., Verstraeten, F., Ham, H., Piepsz, A., & Noel, P. (1989). Regional blood flow in congenital dysphasia: Studies with Technetium-99m HM-PAOSPECT. *Journal of Nueclear Medicine, 30,* 1825–1829.

Deputy, P. N. (1984). The need for description in the study of developmental verbal dyspraxia. *Australian Journal of Human Communication Disorders, 12,* 3–13.

DeRenzi, E., Picczuro, A., & Vignolo, L. A. (1966). Oral apraxia and aphasia. *Cortex, 2,* 50–73.

Doszak, A. L., McNeil, M. R., & Jancosek, E. (1981). *Efficacy of melodic intonation therapy with developmental apraxia of speech.* Paper presented at the annual meeting of the American-Speech-Hearing Association, Los Angeles.

Dunn, L. M., & Dunn, L. M. (1981). *Peabody picture vocabulary test–Revised.* Circle Pines, MN: American Guidance Service.

Dworkin, J. P., Abkarian, G. C., & Johns, D. F. (1988). Apraxia of speech: The effectiveness of a treatment regimen. *Journal of Speech and Hearing Disorders, 53,* 280–294.

Eady, S. J., & Cooper, W. E. (1986). Speech intonation and focus location in matched statements and questions. *Journal of the Acoustical Society of America, 80,* 402–415.

Edwards, M. (1973). Developmental verbal dyspraxia. *British Journal of Disorders of Communication, 8,* 64–70.

Eisenson, J. (1972). *Aphasia in children* (pp. 189–202). New York: Harper & Row.

Ekelmam, B. L. (1981). *Syntactic findings in developmental verbal apraxia.* Paper presented at the annual meeting of the American Speech-Language-Hearing Association, Los Angeles.

Ekelman, B. L., & Aram, D. M. (1983). Syntactic findings in developmental verbal apraxia. *Journal of Communication Disorders, 16,* 237–250.

Ekelman, B. L., & Aram, D. M. (1984). Spoken syntax in children with developmental verbal apraxia. In W. H. Perkins, & J. L. Northern (Eds.), *Seminars in speech and language* (pp. 97–109). New York: Thieme-Stratton.

Elbert, M., & Gierut, J. (1986). *Handbook of clinical phonology.* San Diego: College-Hill Press.

Fawcus, R. (1971). Features of psychological and physiological study of articulatory performance. *British Journal of Disorders of Communication, 6,* 99–106.

Ferry, P. C., Hall, S. M., & Hicks, J. L. (1975). 'Dilapidated' speech: Developmental verbal dyspraxia. *Developmental Medicine and Child Neurology, 17,* 749–756.

Field, E. I. (1977). Response to Dabul & Bollier's "Therapeutic approaches to apraxia." *Journal of Speech and Hearing Disorders, 42,* 311.

Fisher, H. B., & Logemann, J. A. (1971). *The Fisher-Logemann test of articulation competence.* Boston: Houghton-Mifflin.

Fletcher, S. G., & Hasegawa, A. (1983). Speech modification by a deaf child through dynamic orometric modeling and feedback. *Journal of Speech and Hearing Disorders, 48,* 178–185.

Folkins, J. W. (1985). Issues in speech motor control and their relation to the speech of individuals with cleft palate. *Cleft Palate Journal, 22,* 106–122.

Folkins, J. W., & Moon, J. B. (1990). Approaches to the study of speech production. In J. Bardach, & H. Morris, (Eds.), *Multidisciplinary management of cleft lip and palate* (pp. 707–716). Philadelphia: Saunders.

Fromm, D., Abbs, J. H., McNeil, M. R., & Rosenbek, J. C. (1982). Simultaneous perceptual-physiological method for studying apraxia of speech. In R. H.

Brookshire (Ed.), *Proceedings of Clinical Aphasiology Conference* (pp. 251–262). Minneapolis, MN: BRK Publishers.

Fudala, J. B. (1970). *Arizona articulation proficiency scale.* Los Angeles: Western Psychological Services.

Fudula, J. B., & Reynolds, W. M. (1986). *Arizona articulation proficiency scale,* 2nd ed. Los Angeles: Western Psychological Services.

Glasson, C. (1984). Speech timing in children with history of phonologic-phonetic disorders. In W. H. Perkins, & J. L. Northern (Eds.), *Seminars in speech and language* (pp. 85–94). New York: Thieme-Stratton.

Goldman, R., & Fristoe, M. (1969, 1986). *Goldman-Fristoe test of articulation.* Circle Pines, MN: American Guidance Service.

Goldman, R., Fristoe, M., & Woodcock, R. W. (1974). *Test of auditory discrimination.* Circle Pines, MN: American Guidance Service.

Goldwasser, M. K. (1989). *Severe developmental apraxia: A longitudinal case study.* Miniseminar presented at the annual meeting of the American Speech-Language-Hearing Association, St. Louis.

Gorlin, R. J., Cohen, M. M., Jr., & Levin, R. S. (1990). *Syndromes of the head and neck* (3rd ed.). New York: Oxford University Press, Inc.

Greene, M. C. L. (1967). Speechless and backward at three. *British Journal of Disorders of Communication, 2,* 134–145.

Greene, M. C. L. (1983). Development of speech and language: Normal and abnormal. In G. M. English (Ed.), *Otolaryngology, 3,* (pp. 1–23). Philadelphia: Harper & Row.

Grube, M. M., Spiegel, B. B., Buchhop, N. A., & Lloyd, K. L. (1986). Intonational training as a facilitator of intelligibility. *Human Communication Canada, 10*(5), 17–24.

Gubbay, S. S., Ellis, E., Walton, J. N., & Court, S. D. M. (1965). Clumsy children: A study of apraxia and agnostic defects in 21 children. *Brain, 88,* 295–312.

Guyette, T. W., & Diedrich, W. M. (1981). A critical review of developmental apraxia of speech. In N. J. Lass (Ed.), *Speech and language: Advances in basic research and practice* (Vol. 5, pp. 1–49). New York: Academic Press.

Guyette, T. W., & Diedrich, W. M. (1983). A review of the screening test of developmental apraxia of speech. *Language, Speech, and Hearing Services in Schools, 14,* 202–209.

Haaland, K. Y. (1984). The relationship of limb apraxia severity to motor and language deficits. *Brain and Cognition, 3,* 307–316.

Hadden, W. (1891). On certain defects of articulation in children with cases illustrating the results of education of the oral system. *Journal of Mental Science, 37,* 96–105.

Hagen, C. (1987). An approach to the treatment of mild to moderately severe apraxia. *Topics in Language Disorders, 8,* 34–50.

Hall, P. K. (1977). The occurrence of disfluencies in language-disordered school-age children. *Journal of Speech and Hearing Disorders, 42,* 364–369.

Hall, P. K. (1989). The occurrence of developmental apraxia of speech in a mild articulation disorder: A case study. *Journal of Communication Disorders, 22,* 265–276.

Hall, P. K. (1992). At the center of controversy: Developmental apraxia. *American Journal of Speech-Language Pathology: A Journal of Clinical Practice, 1,* 23–25.

Hall, P. K., Hardy, J. C., LaVelle, W. E. (1990). A child with signs of developmental apraxia of speech with whom a palatal lift prosthesis was used to manage palatal dysfunction. *Journal of Speech and Hearing Disorders, 55,* 454–460.

Hall, P. K., & Jordan, L. S. (1987). An assessment of a controlled association task to identify word-finding problems in children. *Language, Speech and Hearing Services in the Schools, 18,* 99–111.

Hall, P. K., & Jordan, L. S. (1992). Use of articulation cuing gestures with children exhibiting developmental apraxia of speech. Poster session presented at the annual meeting of the American Speech-Language-Hearing Association, San Antonio.

Hall, P. K., Robin, D. A., & Jordan, L. S. (1986). *The presence of word-retrieval deficits in developmental verbal apraxia.* Paper presented at the annual meeting of the American Speech-Language-Hearing Association, Detroit.

Hanson, D. M., Jackson, A. W., & Hagerman, R. J. (1986). Speech disturbances (cluttering) in mildly impaired males with Martin-Bell fragile X syndrome. *American Journal of Medical Genetics, 23,* 195–206.

Hardcastle, W. J., MorganBarry, R. A. M., & Clark, C. J. (1987). An instrumental phonetic study of lingual activity in articulation disordered children. *Journal of Speech and Hearing Research, 30,* 171–184.

Hargrove, P. M., Roetzel, K., & Hoodin, R. B. (1989). Modifying the prosody of a language-impaired child. *Language, Speech, and Hearing Services in Schools, 20,* 245–258.

Harlan, N. T. (1984). Treatment approach for a young child evidencing developmental verbal apraxia. *Australian Journal of Human Communication Disorders, 12,* 121–127.

Haynes, S. (1985). Developmental apraxia of speech: Symptoms and treatment. In D. F. Johns (Ed.), *Clinical management of neurogenic communication disorders,* (2nd ed.), (pp. 259–266). Boston: Little, Brown, & Company.

Hejna, R. (1959). *Hejna developmental articulation test.* Ann Arbor, MI: Speech Materials.

Helfrich-Miller, K. R. (1984). Melodic intonation therapy with developmentally apraxic children. In W. H. Perkins & J. L. Northern (Eds.), *Seminars in speech and language* (pp. 119–125). New York: Thieme-Stratton.

Hill, B. (1978). *Verbal dyspraxia in clinical practice.* Carlton, Victoria, Australia: Pitman Publishing Pty. Ltd.

Hixon, T. J., & Hardy, J. C. (1964). Restricted mobility of the speech articulators in cerebral palsy. *Journal of Speech and Hearing Disorders, 29,* 293–306.

Hodson, B. (1986). *Assessment of phonological processes–Revised.* Danville, IL: Interstate Press.

Hodson, B. W., & Paden, E. P. (1983). *Targeting intelligible speech.* Austin, TX: PRO-ED.

Hodson, B. W., & Paden, E. P. (1991). *Targeting intelligible speech.* Austin, TX: PRO-ED.

Horwitz, S. J. (1984). Neurological findings in developmental verbal apraxia. In W. H. Perkins & J. L. Northern (Eds.), *Seminars in speech and language* (pp. 111–118). New York: Thieme-Stratton.

Howard-Peebles, P. N., Stoddard, G. R., & Mims, M. G. (1979). Familial X-linked mental retardation, verbal disability and marker X chromosones. *American Journal of Human Genetics, 31,* 214–222.

Hunter, G. (1975). Childhood apraxia or intra-oral perceptual motor disorder? *Australian Journal of Human Communication Disorders, 3,* 129–140.

Hyland, J., & McNeil, M. R. (1987). The effects of intoning therapy and the speech of a developmentally apraxic adult. In R. Brookshire (Ed.), *Clinical Aphasiology,* (pp. 288–299). Minneapolis, MN: BRK Publishers.

Ingram, T. T. S., & Reid, J. F. (1956). Developmental aphasia observed in a department of child psychiatry. *Archives of Disease in Childhood, 31,* 161–172.

International Communication Learning Institute (1981). *Visual phonics.* Edina, MN: Communication Arts, Inc.

Itoh, M., Sasanuma, S., Ushijuma, T. (1979). Velar movements during speech in a patient with apraxia of speech. *Brain and Language, 7,* 227–239.

Jackson, M. R. F., & Hall, P. K. (1987). *A longitudinal study of articulation characteristics in developmental verbal apraxia.* Paper presented at the annual meeting of the American Speech-Language-Hearing Association, New Orleans.

Jacobs, P. A., Glover, T. W., Mayer, M., Fox, P., Gerrard, J. W., Dunn, H. G., & Herbst, D. S. (1980). X-linked mental retardation: A study of seven families. *American Journal of Medical Genetics, 7,* 471–489.

Jaffe, M. B. (1984). Neurological impairment of speech production: Assessment and treatment. In J. M. Costello (Ed.), *Speech disorders in children* (pp. 157–186). San Diego: College-Hill Press.

Jaffe, M. (1989). Childhood articulatory disorders of neurogenic origin. In M. M. Leahy (Ed.), *Disorders of communication: The science of intervention* (pp. 120–139). New York: Taylor & Francis.

Johns, D. F., & LaPointe, L. L. (1976). Neurogenic disorders of output processing: Apraxia of speech. In H. Whitaker, & H. A. Whitaker (Eds.), *Perspectives in neurolinguisitics and psycholinguisitics* (pp. 161–199). New York: Academic Press.

Johnson, D. J., & Myklebust, H. R. (1967). *Learning disabilities: Educational principles and practices.* New York: Grune & Stratton.

Jordan, L. S. (1988). Gestures for cuing phonemes in verbal apraxia: A case study. Paper presented at the annual meeting of the American Speech-Language-Hearing Association, Boston.

Jordan, L. S. (1991). Treating apraxia of speech. Paper presented at the Midwest Aphasiology Conference, Iowa City.

Jung, J. H. (1989). *Genetic syndromes in communication disorders.* Boston: College-Hill Publications.

Karlin, I. (1958). Speech-and language-handicapped children. *American Journal of Diseases in Children, 95,* 370–376.

Kaufman, N. R., & Hobart, C. J. (1989). *Differential diagnosis of developmental verbal dyspraxia: Normative data.* Paper presented at the annual meeting of the American Speech-Language-Hearing Association, St. Louis.

Kelso, J. A., & Tuller, B. (1981). Toward a theory of apractic syndromes. *Brain and Language, 12,* 224–245.

Kent, R. D. (1976). Models of speech production. In N. J. Lass (Ed.), *Contemporary issues in experimental phonetics* (pp. 79–104). New York: Academic Press.

Kent, R. D., & Lybolt, J. T. (1982). Techniques of therapy based on motor learning theory. In W. H. Perkins (Ed.), *General principles of therapy* (pp. 13–25). New York: Thieme-Stratton.

Khan, L., & Lewis, N. (1986). *Khan-Lewis phonological analysis.* Circle Pines, MN: American Guidance Service.

Klein, E. S. (1987). *Another look at childhood apraxia: It ain't necessarily so.* Miniseminar presented at the annual meeting of the American Speech-Language-Hearing Association, New Orleans.

Klick, S. L. (1985). Adapted cueing technique for use in treatment of dyspraxia. *Language, Speech, and Hearing Services in Schools, 16,* 256–259.

Knuckey, N. W., Apsimon, T. T., & Gubbay, S. S. (1983). Computerized axial tomography in clumsy children with developmental apraxia and agnosia. *Brain Development, 5,* 14–19.

Koay, M. E. T., Morris, R. J., & Walker, V. G. (1989). *Developmental apraxia: Current practices in evaluation and management.* Miniseminar presented at the annual meeting of the American Speech-Language-Hearing Association, St. Louis.

Kornse, D. D., Manni, J. L., Rubenstein, H., & Graziani, L. J. (1981). Developmental apraxia of speech and manual dexterity. *Journal of Communication Disorders, 14,* 321–330.

Krauss, T., & Galloway, H. (1982). Melodic intonation therapy with language delayed apraxic children. *Journal of Music Therapy, 19,* 102–113.

LaPointe, L. L., & Johns, D. F. (1975). Some phonemic characteristics in apraxia of speech. *Journal of Communication Disorders, 8,* 259–269.

Lashley, K. S. (1951). The problem of serial order in behavior. In L. A. Jeffress (Ed.), *Cerebral mechanisms in behavior: The Hixon symposium.* New York: Wiley.

LaVelle, W. E., & Hardy, J. C. (1979). Palatal lift prostheses for treatment of palatopharyngeal incompetence. *Journal of Prosthetic Dentistry, 42,* 308–325.

LaVoi, G. W. (1986). *A comparative analysis of selected variables in apraxic and nonapraxic children.* Paper presented at the annual meeting of the American Speech-Language-Hearing Association, Detroit.

Lee, L. (1971). *Northwestern syntax screening test.* Evanston, IL: Northwestern University Press.

Lesny, I. A. (1980). Developmental dyspraxia-dysgnosia as a cause of congenital children's clumsiness. *Brain Development, 2,* 69–71.

Lewis, B. A. (1989). *Family pedigrees of phonology disordered children.* Paper presented at the annual meeting of the American Speech-Language-Hearing Association, St.Louis.

Lewis, B. A. (1990). A familial phonological disorder: Four pedigrees. *Journal of Speech and Hearing Disorders, 55,* 160–170.

Lewis, B. A., Ekelman, B. L., & Aram, D. M. (1989). A familial study of severe phonological disorders. *Journal of Speech and Hearing Research, 32,* 713–724.

Lewis, N., & Greenbaum, M. (1985). *A phonological approach to remediation for three developmentally apraxic children.* Paper presented at the annual meeting of the American Speech-Language-Hearing Association, Washington, DC.

Liepmann, H. (1900). Das krankheitsbild der apraxie (motorischen asymbolie) auf grund eines falles von einseitigen apraxie. *Monatschrift fur Psychiatrie und Neurologie, 8,* 15–40.

Lohr, F. E. (1978). The nonverbal apraxic child: Definition, evaluation, and therapy. *Western Michigan University Journal of Speech, Language, and Hearing, 15,* 3–6.

Love, R. J. (1992). *Childhood motor speech disability.* New York: Merrill Macmillan Publishing Company.

Love, R. J., & Fitzgerald, M. (1984). Is the diagnosis of developmental apraxia of speech valid? *Australian Journal of Human Communication Disorders, 12,* 71–82.

Lucas, D. R., Weiss, A. L., & Hall, P. K. (1989). *Response to communicative failure in children with different communication disorders.* Paper presented at the annual meeting of the American Speech-Language-Hearing Association, St. Louis.

Lucas, D. R., Weiss, A. L., & Hall, P. K. (In Press). Assessing referential communication skills: The use of a non-standardized assessment procedure. *Journal of Childhood Communication Disorders.*

Luchsinger, R., & Arnold, G. E. (1965). *Voice-speech-language clinical communicology: Its physiology and pathology.* Belmont, CA: Wadsworth.

Macaluso-Haynes, S. (1978). Developmental apraxia of speech: Symptoms and treatment. In D. F. Johns (Ed.), *Clinical management of neurogenic communication disorders,* (pp. 243–250). Boston: Little, Brown, & Company.

Madison, L. S., George, C., & Moeschler, J. B. (1986). Cognitive functioning in the fragile X syndrome: A study of intellectual, memory and communication skills. *Journal of Mental Deficiency Research, 30,* 129–148.

Marquardt, T. P., Dunn, C., & Davis, B. (1985). Apraxia of speech in children. In J. K. Darby (Ed.), *Speech and language evaluation in neurology: Childhood disorders* (pp. 113–129). Needham Heights, MA: Allyn & Bacon.

Marquardt, T. P., Reinhart, J. B., & Peterson, H. A. (1979). Markedness analysis of phonemic substitution errors in apraxia of speech. *Journal of Communication Disorders, 12,* 481–494.

Marquardt, T. P., & Sussman, H. M. (1991). Developmental apraxia of speech: Theory and practice. In D. Vogel & M. P. Cannito (Eds.), *Treating disordered speech motor control* (pp. 341–390). Austin, TX: PRO-ED.

Marshall, J. C. (1982). What is a symptom-complex? In M. Arbib, D. Caplan, & J. Marshall (Eds.), *Neural models of language processes* (pp. 389–409). New York: Academic Press.

Marteniuk, R. G. (1986). Information processes in movement learning: Capacity and structural interference effects. *Journal of Motor Behavior, 18,* 55–75.

Martin, A. D. (1974). Some objections to the term 'apraxia of speech.' *Journal of Speech and Hearing Disorders, 39,* 53–64.

Mattis, S., French, J. H., & Rapin, I. (1975). Dyslexia in children and young adults: Three independent neuropsychological syndromes. *Developmental Medicine and Child Neurology, 17,* 150–163.

McCabe, R. B., & Bradley, D. P. (1975). Systematic multiple phonemic approach to articulation therapy. *Acta Symbolica, 6,* 1–18.

McCarthy, D. (1972). *McCarthy scales of children's abilities.* New York: Psychological Corporation.

McCauley, R. J., & Swisher, L. (1984a). Psychometric review of language and articulation tests for preschool children. *Journal of Speech and Hearing Disorders, 49,* 34–42.

McCauley, R. J., & Swisher, L. (1984b). Use and misuse of norm-referenced tests in clinical assessment: A hypothetical case. *Journal of Speech and Hearing Disorders, 49,* 338–348.

McClean, M. D., Buekelman, D. R., & Yorkston, K. M. (1987). Speech-muscle visuomotor tracking in dysarthric and nonimpaired speakers. *Journal of Speech and Hearing Research, 30,* 276–282.

McCormick, L., & Shane, H. (1990). Communication system options for students who are nonspeaking. In L. McCormick & R. L. Schiefelbusch (Eds.), *Early Language Intervention* (pp. 428–471). Columbus, OH: Merrill Publishing Company.

McCroskey, J. C. (1984). *Avoiding communication: Shyness, reticence and communication apprehension.* Beverly Hills: Sage Publications.

McDonald, E. T. (1964). *Articulation testing and treatment: A sensory-motor approach.* Pittsburgh: Stanwix House.

McGinnis, M. A. (1963). *Aphasic children.* Washington, DC: Alexander Graham Bell Association for the Deaf.

McGinnis, M. A. (1988). Aphasic children: Identification and education by the Association Method. In *Teaching aphasic children: The instructional methods of Barry and McGinnis* (pp. 63–226). Austin, TX: PRO-ED.

McGinnis, M. A., Kleffner, F. R., & Goldstein, R. (1956). Teaching aphasic children. *Volta Review, 58,* 239–244.

McKusick, V. A. (1990). *Mendelian inheritance in man: Catalog of autosomal dominant, autosomal recessive, and X-linked phenotypes* (9th ed). Baltimore: Johns Hopkins University Press.

McLaughlin, J. F., & Kriegsmann, E. (1980). Developmental dyspraxia in a family with X-linked mental retardation (Renpenning Syndrome). *Developmental Medicine and Child Neurology, 22,* 84–92.

McNeil, M. R., Weismer, G., Adams, S., & Mulligan, M. (1990). Oral structure nonspeech motor control in normal, dysarthric, aphasic, and apraxic speakers: Isometric force and static position control. *Journal of Speech and Hearing Research, 33,* 255–268.

McReynolds, L. V., & Kearns, K. P. (1983). *Single-subject experimental designs in communicative disorders.* Austin, TX: PRO-ED.

Milloy, N., & Summers, L. (1989). Six years on—do claims still hold? Four children reassessed on a procedure to identify developmental articulatory dyspraxia. *Child Language Teaching and Therapy, 5,* 287–303.

Minskoff, E. H. (1980a). Teaching approach for developing nonverbal skills in students with social perception deficits: Part 1. The basic approach and body language clues. *Journal of Learning Disabilities, 13,* 118–124.

Minskoff, E. H. (1980b). Teaching approach for developing nonverbal skills in students with social perception deficits. Part II. Proxemic, vocalic, and artifactual cues. *Journal of Learning Disabilities, 13,* 203–208.

Mlcoch, A. G., & Noll, J. D. (1980). Speech production models as related to the concept of apraxia of speech. In N. J. Lass (Ed.), *Speech and language: Advances in basic research and practice,* Vol. 4, (pp. 201–239). New York: Academic Press.

Mlcoch, A. G., & Square, P. A. (1984). Apraxia of speech: Articulatory and perceptual factors. In N. Lass (Ed.), *Speech and language: Advances in basic research and practice,* Vol. 10, (pp. 1–57). New York: Academic Press.

Monson, R., Moog, J. S., & Geers, A. E. (1988). *CID picture SPINE: Speech intelligiblity evaluation.* St. Louis, MO: Central Institute for the Deaf.

Moon, J. B. (1993). Evaluation of velopharyngeal closure. In K. Moller & C. Starr (Eds.), *Cleft Palate: Interdisciplinary issues and treatment* (pp.251–306). Austin, TX: PRO-ED.

Moon, J. B., Robin, D. A., Zebrowski, P., & Folkins, J. W. (1991). *Visual motor tracking: A method for evaluating speech motor control.* Paper presented at the annual meeting of the American Speech-Language-Hearing Association, Atlanta.

MorganBarry, R. M. (1989). EPG from square one: An overview of electropalatography as an aid to therapy. *Clinical Linguistics & Phonetics, 3,* 81–91.

Morley, M. E. (1957). *The development and disorders of speech in childhood.* London, England: Livingstone.

Morley, M. E. (1959). Defects of articulation. *Folia Phoniatrica, 11,* 65–124.

Morley, M. E. (1965). *The development and disorders of speech in childhood* (2nd ed.). Baltimore: Williams and Wilkins Company.

Morley, M. E. (1972). *The development and disorders of speech in childhood* (3rd ed.). London, England: Livingstone.

Morley, M. E., Court, D., & Miller, H. (1954). Developmental dysarthria. *British Medical Journal, 1,* 8–10.

Morley, M., Court, D., Miller, H., & Garside, R. F. (1955). Delayed speech and developmental aphasia. *British Medical Journal, 2,* 463–467.

Morley, M. E., & Fox, J. (1969). Disorders of articulation: Theory and therapy. *British Journal of Disorders of Communication, 4,* 151–165.

Murdoch, B. E., Porter, S., Younger, R., & Ozanne, A. (1984). Behaviors identified by South Australian clinicians as differentially diagnostic of developmental dyspraxia. *Australian Journal of Human Communication Disorders, 12,* 55–70.

Nelson, C. D., Waggoner, D. D., Donnell, G. N., Tuerck, J. M., & Buist, N. R. (1991). Verbal dyspraxia in treated galactosemia. *Pediatrics, 88,* 346–350.

Newell, K., Sanborn, B., & Hagerman, R. J. (1983). Speech and language dysfunction in the fragile X syndrome. In R. J. Hagerman & P. McBogg (Eds.), *The fragile X syndrome: Diagnosis, biochemistry and intervention* (pp. 175–239). Dillon, CO: Spectra Publishing.

Nicolosi, L., Harryman, E., & Kreschek, J. (1983). *Terminology of communication disorders: Speech, language, and hearing.* Baltimore: Williams & Wilkins.

Oberle, I., Rousseau, F., Heitz, D., Kretz, C., Devys, D., Hanauer, A., Boue, J., Bertheas, M. F., & Mandel, J. L. (1991). Instability of a 550-base pair DNA segment and abnormal methylatian in fragile X syndrome. *Science, 252,* 1097–1102.

Orton, S. T. (1937). *Reading, writing and speech problems in children.* New York: W. W. Norton.

Palmer, M. F., Wurth, C. W., & Kincholoe, J. W. (1964). The incidence of lingual apraxia and agnosia in "functional" disorders of articulation. *Cerebral Palsy Review, 25,* 7–9.

Panagos, J. M., & Bobokoff, K. (1984). Beliefs about developmental apraxia of speech. *Australian Journal of Human Communication Disorders, 12,* 39–53.

Pannbacker, M. (1988). Management strategies for developmental apraxia of speech: A review of literature. *Journal of Communication Disorders, 21,* 363–371.

Parsons, C. L. (1984). A comparison of phonological processes used by developmentally verbal dyspraxic children and non-dyspraxic phonologically impaired children. *Australian Journal of Human Communication Disorders, 12,* 93–107.

Paul, R., Cohen, D. J., Breg, W. R., Watson, M., & Herman, S. (1984). Fragile X syndrome: Its relations to speech and language disorders. *Journal of Speech and Hearing Disorders, 49,* 328–332.

Paul, R., Dykens, E., Leckman, J. F., Watson, M., Breg, W. R., & Cohen, D. J. (1987). A comparison of language characteristics of mentally retarded adults with fragile X syndrome and those with nonspecific mental retardation. *Journal of Autism and Developmental Disabilities, 17*(4), 457–468.

Pendergast, K., Dickey, S. E., Selmar, J. W., & Soder, A. L. (1969). *Photo articulation test.* Danville, IL: The Interstate Printers and Publishers.

Perkins, W. H. (1984). Forward. In W. H. Perkins & J. L. Northern (Eds.), *Seminars in speech and language* (unnumbered pages). New York: Thieme-Stratton.

Pollock, K. E., & Hall, P. K. (1991). An analysis of vowel misarticulations in five children with developmental apraxia of speech. *Clinical Linguistics and Phonetics, 5,* 207–224.

Pollock, K. E., & Keiser, N. J. (1990). An examination of vowel errors in phonologically disordered children. *Clinical Linguistics and Phonetics, 4,* 161–178.

Povel, D. J., & Wansink, M. (1986). A computer-controlled vowel corrector for the hearing impaired. *Journal of Speech and Hearing Research, 29,* 99–105.

Prichard, C. L., Tekieli, M. E., & Kozup, J. M. (1979). Developmental apraxia: Diagnostic considerations. *Journal of Communication Disorders, 12,* 337–348.

Rapin, I., & Allen, D. A. (1981). Progress toward a nosology of developmental dysphasia. In Y. Fukuyama, M. Arima, K. Maekawa, & K. Yamaguchi (Eds.), *Child Neurology* (pp. 25–35), International Congress Series, Proceedings of the IYDP Commerative International Symposium on Developmental Disabilities, Tokyo.

Rapin, I., & Wilson, B. C. (1978). Children with developmental langauage disability: Neurological aspects and assessment. In M. A. Wyke (Ed.), *Developmental dysphasia* (pp. 13–41). New York: Academic Press.

Riess, D. (1987). *Accuracy of normal and developmentally verbal apraxic children in tasks of speech diadochokinesis.* Unpublished honors thesis. University of Iowa, Iowa City, IA.

Riley, G. D. (1984). Developmental verbal dyspraxia: A clinical perspective. *Australian Journal of Human Communication Disorders, 12,* 83–91.

Robin, D. A. (1992). Developmental apraxia of speech: Just another motor problem. *American Journal of Speech-Language Pathology: A Journal of Clinical Practice, 1,* 19–22.

Robin, D. A., Bean, C., & Folkins, J. W. (1989). Lip movement in apraxia of speech. *Journal of Speech and Hearing Research, 32,* 512–523.

Robin, D. A., Hall, P. K., & Jordan, L. S. (1986). *Auditory processing deficits in developmental verbal apraxia.* Paper presented at the annual meeting of the American Speech-Language-Hearing Association, Detroit.

Robin, D. A., Hall, P. K., & Jordan, L. S. (1987). *Prosodic impairment in developmental verbal apraxia.* Paper presented at the annual meeting of the American Speech-Language-Hearing Association, New Orleans.

Robin, D. A., Hall, P. K., Jordan, L. S., & Gordan, A. J. (1991). *Developmentally apraxic speakers' stress production: Perceptual and acoustic analyses.* Paper presented at the annual meeting of the American Speech-Language-Hearing Association, Atlanta.

Robin, D. A., Klouda, G. V., & Hug, L. N. (1991). Neurogenic disorders of prosody. In M. P. Cannito & D. Vogel (Eds.), *Treating disordered speech motor control: For clinicians by clinicians* (pp. 241–271). Austin, TX: PRO-ED.

Robin, D. A., & McNeil, M. R. (1992). The use of signal detection theory to evaluate aphasia diagnostic accuracy and bias. *Clinical Aphasiology, 21,* 193–205.

Robin, D. A., & Royer, F. L. (1987). Auditory temporal processing: Two-tone flutter fusion and a model of temporal integration. *Journal of the Acoustical Society of America, 82,* 1207–1217.

Robin, D. A., Tomblin, J. B., Kearney, A., & Hug, L. N. (1989). Auditory temporal pattern learning in children with speech and language impairments. *Brain and Language, 36,* 604–613.

Robin, D. A., Tranel, D., & Damasio, H. (1990). Auditory perception of temporal and spectral events in patients with focal left and right cerebral lesions. *Brain and Language, 39,* 539–555.

Roe, V., & Milisen, R. (1942). The effect of maturation upon defective articulation in elementary grades. *Journal of Speech Disorders, 7,* 37–42.

Rood, M. (1954). Neurophysiological reactions as a basis for physical therapy. *Physical Therapy Review, 34,* 444–449.

Rosenbek, J. C. (1985). Treating apraxia of speech. In D. F. Johns (Ed.), *Clinical management of neurogenic communication disorders* (2nd ed.), (pp. 267–312). Boston: Little, Brown, & Company.

Rosenbek, J. C., Hansen, R., Baughman, C. H., & Lemme, M. (1974). Treatment of developmental apraxia of speech: A case study. *Language, Speech, Hearing Services in Schools, 5,* 13–22.

Rosenbek, J. C., Kent, R. D., & LaPointe, L. L. (1984). Apraxia of speech: An overview and some perspectives. In J. C. Rosenbek, M. R. McNeil, & A. E. Aronson (Eds.), *Apraxia of Speech: Physiology, acoustics, linguistics, management* (pp. 1–72). San Diego: College-Hill Press.

Rosenbek, J. C., & Wertz, R. T. (1972). A review of fifty cases of developmental apraxia of speech. *Language, Speech, and Hearing Services in Schools, 5,* 23–33.

Roy, E. A. (1978). Apraxia: A new look at an old syndrome. *Journal of Human Movement Studies, 4,* 191–210.

Salmoni, A. W., Schmidt, R. A., & Walter, C. B. (1984). Knowledge of results and motor learning: A review and critical reappraisal. *Psychological Bulletin, 95,* 355–386.

Salvia, J., & Ysseldyke, J. E. (1991). *Assessment* (5th ed.). Boston: Houghton-Mifflin Company.

Sands, E. S., Freeman, F. J., & Harris, K. S. (1978). Progressive changes in articulatory patterns in verbal apraxia: A longitudinal study. *Brain and Language, 6,* 97–105.

Scharfenaker, S. K. (1990). The fragile X syndrome. *Journal of the American Speech-Language-Hearing Association, 32,* September, 45–47.

Scherer, K. R. (1986). Vocal affect expression: A review and a model for future research. *Psychological Bulletin, 99,* 143–165.

Schmidt, R. A. (1975). A schema theory of discrete motor learning. *Psychological Review, 82,* 225–260.

Schmidt, R. A. (1988). *Motor control and learning: A behavioral emphasis* (2nd. ed.). Champaign, IL: Human Kinetics Publishers, Inc.

Schumacher, J. G., McNeil, M. R., Vetter, D. K., & Yoder, D. E. (1984). *Efficacy of treatment: Melodic intonation therapy with developmentally apraxic children.* Paper presented at the annual meeting of the American Speech-Language-Hearing Association, San Fransisco.

Selkirk, E. O. (1984). *Phonology and syntax: The relation between sound and structure.* Cambridge, MA: MIT Press.

Semjen, A. (1977). From motor learning to sensorimotor skill acquisition. *Journal of Human Movement Studies, 3,* 182–191.

Shapiro, D. C., & Schmidt, R. A. (1982). The schema theory: Recent evidence and developmental implications. In J. A. S. Kelso & J. E. Clark (Eds.), *The development of movement control and coordination* (pp. 113–150). New York: Wiley.

Shea, J. B., & Upton, G. (1976). The effects on skill acquisition of an interpolated motor short-term memory task during the KR-delay interval. *Journal of Motor Behavior, 8,* 277–281.

Shelton, I. K., & Graves, M. M. (1985). Use of visual techniques in therapy for devlopmental apraxia of speech. *Language, Speech, and Hearing Services in Schools, 16,* 129–131.

Shuster, L. I., Ruscello, D. M., & Haines, K. B. (1989). *Acoustic patterns of developmental apraxia of speech.* Paper presented at the annual meeting of the American Speech-Language-Hearing Association, St. Louis.

Silverman, F. H. (1980). *Communication for the speechless.* Englewood Cliffs, NJ: Prentice Hall.

Snowling, M., & Stackhouse, J. (1983). Spelling performance of children with developmental verbal dyspraxia. *Developmental Medicine & Child Neurology, 25,* 430–437.

Snyder, D. R., Marquardt, T. P., & Peterson, H. A. (1977). Syntactical aspects of developmental apraxia. *Human Communication, 2,* 151–158.

Sommers, R. K. (1983). *Articulation disorders.* Englewood Cliffs, NJ: Prentice-Hall.

Sparks, R. W., & Deck, J. W. (1986). Melodic intonation therapy. In R. Chapey (Ed.). *Language intervention strategies in adult aphasia* (pp. 320–332). Baltimore: Williams & Wilkins.

Sparks, R. W., Helm, N., & Albert, M. (1974). Aphasia rehabilitation resulting from Melodic intonation therapy. *Cortex, 10,* 303–316.

Sparks, R., & Holland, A. (1976). Method: Melodic intonation therapy for aphasia. *Journal of Speech and Hearing Disorders, 41,* 287–297.

Spriestersbach, D.C., Morris, H. L., & Darley, F. L. (1978). Examination of the speech mechanism. In F. L. Darley & D. C. Spriestersbach (Eds.), *Diagnostic methods in speech pathology* (pp. 322–345). New York: Harper & Row.

Sternberg, S., Monsell, S., Knoll, R. L., & Wright, C. E. (1978). The latency duration of rapid movement sequences: Comparisons of speech and typewriting. In G. E. Stelmach (Ed.), *Information processing in motor control and learning* (pp. 117–152). New York: Academic Press.

Stinchfield, S. M., & Young, E. H. (1938). *Children with delayed or defective speech.* Palo Alto, CA: Stanford University Press.

Stockmeyer, A. (1967). An interpretation of the approach of Rood to the treatment of neuromuscular dysfunction. *American Journal of Physical Medicine, 46,* 900–956.

Stoel-Gammon, C., & Dunn, C. (1985). *Normal and disordered phonology in children.* Baltimore: University Park Press.

Strand, E. A., Brown, J. J., & Moss, M. (1989). *Developmental apraxia of speech: A treatment efficacy study.* Paper presented at the annual meeting of the American Speech-Language-Hearing Association, St. Louis.

Streng, A. (1955). *Hearing therapy for children.* New York: Grune & Stratton.

Swanson, C. (1987). *An analysis of grammatical morpheme errors in children with developmental verbal apraxia.* Unpublished honors thesis. University of Iowa, Iowa City, IA.

Swets, J. A., & Pickett, R. M. (1982). *Evaluation of diagnostic systems: Methods from signal detection theory.* New York: Academic Press.

Templin, M. C. (1957). *Certain language skills in children* (Institute of Child Welfare Monograph Series, Number 26). Minneapolis: University of Minnesota Press.

Templin, M., & Darley, F. (1969). *The Templin-Darley tests of articulation.* Iowa City, IA: University of Iowa Bureau of Educational Research and Service.

Thompson, C. K. (1988). Articulation disorders in the child with neurogenic pathology. In N. J. Lass, L. V. McReynolds, J. L. Northern, & D. E. Yoder (Eds.), *Handbook of Speech-Language Pathology and Audiology* (pp. 548–591). Philadelphia: B. C. Decker.

Tomblin, J. B. (1991). Inquiries into the genetics of specific language impairment. (Keynote talk). American Speech-Language-Hearing Association Research Conference, Atlanta.

Towne, R. L., & Crary, M. A. (1982). *Syntagmatic distance as a phonological variable in developmental verbal dyspraxia.* Paper presented at the annual meeting of the American Speech-Language-Hearing Association, Toronto.

Trost-Cardamone, J. E. (1986). Effects of velopharyngeal incompetence on speech. *Journal of Childhood Communication Disorders, 10,* 31–49.

Turner, G., Daniel, A., & Frost, M. (1980). X-linked mental retardation, macro or chidism and the Xa27 fragile site. *Journal of Pediatrics, 96,* 836–841.

Vaughn, G. R., & Clark, R. M. (1979). *Speech facilitation: Extraoral and intraoral stimulation technique for improvement of articulation skills.* Springfield, IL: Charles C. Thomas Publisher.

Wade, M. G. (1982). Timing behavior in children. In J. A. Scott Kelso & J. E. Clark (Eds.), *The development of movement control and coordination* (pp. 239–252). New York: John Wiley & Sons, LTD.

Walton, J. N., Ellis, E., & Court, S. D. M. (1962). Clumsy children: Developmental apraxia and agnosia. *Brain, 85,* 603–612.

Wechsler, D. (1974). *Wechsler intelligence scale for children.* New York: Psychological Corporation.

Weiner, D. S. (1960). The perceptual level functioning of dysphasic children. *Cortex, 5,* 440–457.

Weiss, C. E., Gordon, M. E., & Lillywhite, H. S. (1987). *Clinical management of articulatory and phonologic disorders* (pp. 259–269). Baltimore: Williams & Wilkins.

Wertz, R. T., LaPointe, L. L., & Rosenbek, J. C. (1984). *Apraxia of speech in adults: The disorder and its management.* New York: Grune & Stratton.

Williams, R., Ingham, R. J., & Rosenthal, J. (1981). A further analysis for developmental apraxia of speech in children with defective articulation. *Journal of Speech and Hearing Research, 24,* 496–506.

Williams, C. E., & Stevens, K. N. (1972). Emotions and speech: Some acoustical correlates. *Journal of the Acoustical Society of America, 52,* 1238–1250.

Wingfield, A., Lombardi, L., & Sokol, S. (1984). Prosodic features and the intelligibility of accelerated speech: Syntactic versus periodic segmentation. *Journal of Speech and Hearing Research, 27,* 128–134.

Wiznitzer, M., Rapin, I., & Allen, D. (1986). *Motor function in school-age children with developmental language disorders.* Program and abstract of paper presented at the annual meeting of the Child Neurology Society, Boston.

Wode, H. (1980). Grammatic intonation in child language. In L. R. Waugh & C. H. van Schooneveld (Eds.), *The melody of language* (pp. 331–345). Baltimore: University Park Press.

Wolk, L. (1984). Phonological and neuroanatomical findings in three cases with apraxia of speech. *South African Journal of Communication Disorders, 31,* 36–47.

Woodruff, M. K. (1988). *A study of the presence of variability in developmental apraxia of speech.* Unpublished honors thesis. University of Iowa, Iowa City, IA.

Worster-Draught, C. (1953). Report: Failure in normal language development of neurological origin. *Folia Phoniatrica, 5,* 130–146.

Yorkston, K. M., & Beukelman, D. R. (1984). *Assessment of intelligibility of dysarthric speech.* Tigard, OR: C. C. Publications.

Yoss, K. A., & Darley, F. L. (1974a). Developmental apraxia of speech in children with defective articulation. *Journal of Speech and Hearing Research, 17,* 399–416.

Yoss, K. A., & Darley, F. L. (1974b). Therapy in developmental apraxia of speech. *Language, Speech, and Hearing Services in Schools, 5,* 23–31.

Yost, W. A., & Nielsen, D. W. (1977). *Fundamentals of hearing: An introduction.* New York: Holt, Rinehart & Winston.

Young, E. H., & Hawk, S. S. (1955). *Motokinesthetic speech training.* Stanford, CA: Stanford University Press.

Yu, S., Pritchard, M., Kremer, E., Lynch, M., Nancarrow, J., Baker, E., Holman, K., Mulley, J. C., Warren, S. T., Schlessinger, D., Sutherland, G. R., & Richards, R. I. (1991). Fragile X genotype characterized by an unstable region of DNA. *Science, 252,* 1179–1181.

Author Index

201

Subject Index